Self-Assessment Color Review

# Small Animal Neurology

Simon J. Wheeler
BVSc, PhD, MRCVS
Diplomate, European College of
Veterinary Neurology
Royal Veterinary College
University of London

William B. Thomas
DVM, MS
Diplomate, American College of Veterinary Internal
Medicine (Neurology)
College of Veterinary Medicine
University of Tennessee, Knoxville

Manson Publishing/The Veterinary Press

# Acknowledgements

The authors are grateful to Dr Andrew Hopkins for reviewing the manuscript and making many useful suggestions.

The following colleagues loaned illustrations, for which we are grateful: Drs Robert DeNovo, Susan Orosz, Robert Seleer, and Robert Shull.

The illustrations in Question **147** (MRI) are from Thomas WB, Wheeler SJ, Kramer R, Kornegay JN. Magnetic resonance imaging features of primary brain tumors in dogs. *Vet Radiol & Ultrasound* 1996; 37: 20-27, and are reproduced with permission.

The line drawings with Answers **1, 110** and **154** are redrawn, with permission, from *Manual of Small Animal Neurology* (ed. SJ Wheeler), BSAVA, Cheltenham, 1995. The drawing with Answer **82** is redrawn, with permission, from *Small Animal Spinal Disorders* (SJ Wheeler and NJH Sharp), Mosby-Wolfe, London, 1994.

Finally, we should like to acknowledge our colleagues who acted as an inspiration and a continued stimulus to 'keep on our toes': Drs Rod Bagley, Laurent Cauzinille, Sue Fitzmaurice, Andrew Hopkins, Joe Kornegay, Rick LeCouteur, Alistair McVey, Scott Plummer, Clare Rusbridge, Ron Schueler, Robert Selcer, Nick Sharp, and Elizabeth Shull.

Second impression 2001
Copyright © 1996 Manson Publishing Ltd
ISBN 1-874545-33-2

All rights reserved. No part of this publication may be reproduced, stored in a retrieval system or transmitted in any form or by any means without the written permission of the copyright holder or in accordance with the provisions of the Copyright Act 1956 (as amended), or under the terms of any licence permitting limited copying issued by the Copyright Licensing Agency, 33–34 Alfred Place, London WC1E 7DP.

Any person who does any unauthorised act in relation to this publication may be liable to criminal prosecution and civil claims for damages.

A CIP catalogue record for this book is available from the British Library.

For full details of all Manson Publishing Ltd titles please write to Manson Publishing Ltd, 73 Corringham Road, London NW11 7DL, UK.

Design and layout: Patrick Daly
Colour separations by: Reed Reprographics, Ipswich, UK
Printed by: Grafos SA, Barcelona, Spain

# Glossary of acronyms

| | |
|---|---|
| ACh | Acetylcholine |
| AChR | Acetylcholine receptor |
| ALT | Alanine aminotransferase |
| AP | Alkaline phosphatase |
| BAEP | Brainstem auditory evoked potential |
| BUN | Blood urea nitrogen |
| CK | Creatine kinase |
| CNS | Central nervous system |
| CP | Conscious proprioception |
| CT | Computed tomography |
| ELISA | Enzyme-linked immunosorbent assay |
| EMG | Electromyogram |
| ERG | Electroretinogram |
| FeLV | Feline leukaemia virus |
| FIP | Feline infectious peritonitis |
| FIV | Feline immunodeficiency virus |
| GI | Gastrointestinal |
| GME | Granulomatous meningoencephalomyelitis |
| ICP | Intracranial pressure |
| LMN | Lower motor neuron |
| MG | Myasthenia gravis |
| MRI | Magnetic resonance imaging |
| PCV | Packed cell volume (haematocrit) |
| PLR | Pupillary light reflex |
| SARD | Sudden acquired retinal degeneration |
| UMN | Upper motor neuron |
| UTI | Urinary tract infection |
| WBC | White blood cells |

# Preface

This book is a collection of illustrated questions and answers covering many aspects of small animal neurology. The book aims to question and also to educate the reader. The questions vary in difficulty, with the more basic aimed at veterinary students and the more complex at the more experienced clinician. The questions are mixed randomly throughout the book.
The description of neurological findings is given in the form used by most teachers of neurology and as presented in the standard texts. The reader is encouraged to refer to these for descriptions of the neurological examination and its interpretation (see below). In particular, the following classification of reflex and other findings of the neurological examination is used:

| | |
|---|---|
| Absent | 0 |
| Reduced | +1 |
| Normal | +2 |
| Increased | +3 |
| Clonus | +4 |

The anatomical terms given in the *Nomina Anatomica Veterinaria* are largely used throughout the book. Some of these terms may be unfamiliar to many readers, and alternatives are given where appropriate.
References and further reading are indicated at the end of answers, as appropriate.

## Further reading

DeLahunta A. *Veterinary Neuroanatomy and Clinical Neurology*, 2nd edn. Philadelphia: Saunders, 1983.
*Nomina Anatomica Veterinaria*. Ithaca, NY: World Association of Veterinary Anatomists, 1983.
Oliver JE, Hoerlein BF, Mayhew IG (eds). *Veterinary Neurology*. Philadelphia: Saunders, 1987.
Wheeler SJ (ed). *Manual of Small Animal Neurology*, 2nd edn. Cheltenham: BSAVA, 1995.

# 1 & 2: Questions

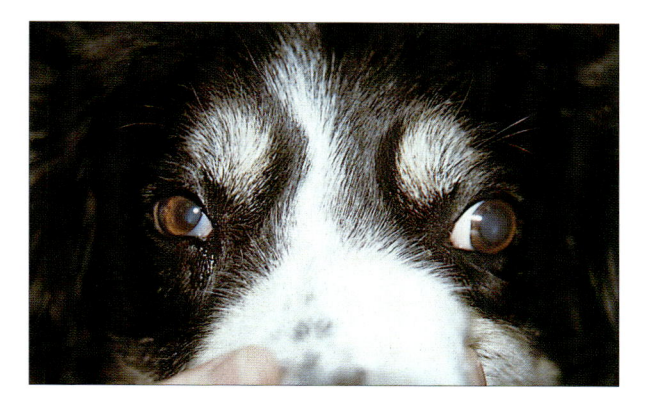

**1** i. What ophthalmological disorder does this dog have?
ii. Where could the lesion be?
iii. What pharmacological test may help determine the location of the lesion?

**2** A five-year-old Dachshund is presented with acute paraplegia, which occurred 24 hours previously. Neurological examination indicates a lesion in the T3–L3 spinal cord segments. The panniculus reflex indicates a T12/T13 lesion. There is no deep pain sensation in the pelvic limbs. There is degenerative disc disease, and myelography indicates an extradural lesion at L2/L3.
i. What is the most likely diagnosis?
ii. What are the treatment options?
iii. Which is the most appropriate method of treatment?
iv. What is the prognosis?

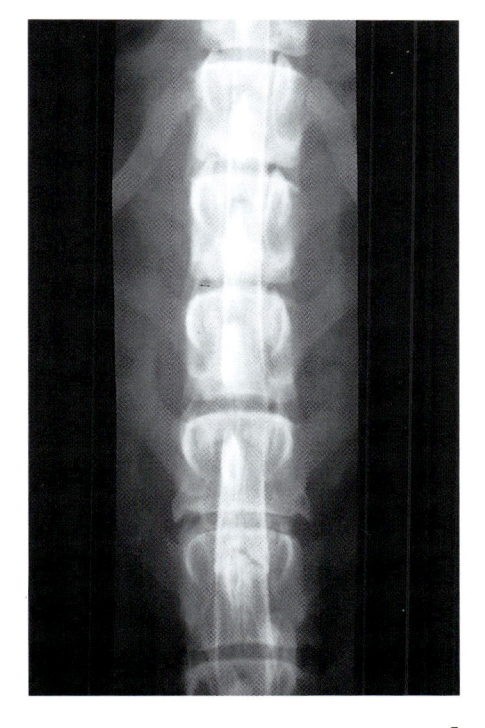

# 1 & 2: Answers

**1 i.** Horner's syndrome – interference with sympathetic nervous supply to the eye.
**ii.** The lesion localisation is illustrated below (see also **A154**).

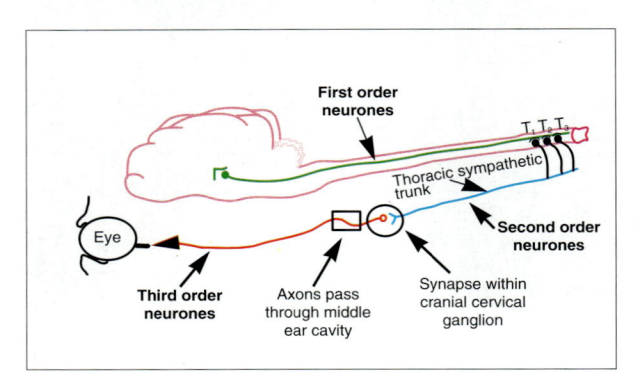

**iii.** 10% phenylephrine is administered topically to both eyes and the time taken for the pupils to dilate is noted. The pupil of a normal eye, or one with a first order Horner's syndrome, will dilate in 60–90 minutes. Eyes with second-order lesions dilate in approximately 45 minutes, and those with third-order lesions in approximately 20 minutes.

### Reference
Petersen-Jones SM. Abnormalities of eyes and vision. In: Wheeler SJ (ed). *Manual of Small Animal Neurology*, 2nd edn. Cheltenham: BSAVA, 1995: 152–154.

**2 i.** Disc extrusion.
**ii.** Treatment may be either non-surgical or surgical. Non-surgical treatment involves strict cage rest, possibly accompanied by analgesics. Surgical treatments include fenestration (where disc material is removed from the intervertebral spaces, but not the vertebral canal) or decompression, usually via a hemilaminectomy. In the latter operation disc material is removed from the vertebral canal, thus decompressing the spinal cord. In association with either treatment method, use of high-dose methylprednisolone sodium succinate may be beneficial within eight hours of the injury.
**iii.** Surgical decompression via hemilaminectomy.
**iv.** If performed within 48 hours of the onset of paralysis, decompression will provide a significantly better prognosis (approximately 50% of patients will recover) than fenestration or non-surgical treatment (where the recovery rate is around 7%). However, if decompressive surgery is delayed beyond 48 hours, the benefits are lost. Occasionally, patients will die as a consequence of this disease, usually as a result of progressive myelomalacia.

### Reference
Wheeler SJ, Sharp NJH. *Small Animal Spinal Disorders*. London: Mosby-Wolfe, 1994: 88.

# 3–5: Questions

3  The dog described in Q2 is treated conservatively. What are the most important considerations in treatment and nursing?

4  An 8-year-old Standard poodle is presented with severe neck pain and a mild asymmetrical tetraparesis. The myelogram (**right**) and a transverse computed tomography (CT) image through mid-C4 are shown (**below right**). Describe and interpret the radiological features.

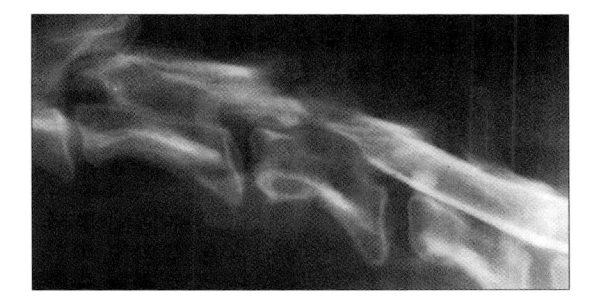

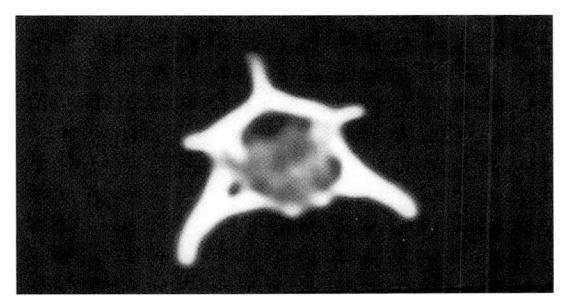

5  The radiograph is of a one-year-old Persian cat with a three month duration of sneezing and a recent onset of a head tilt to the left. Interpret the radiograph.

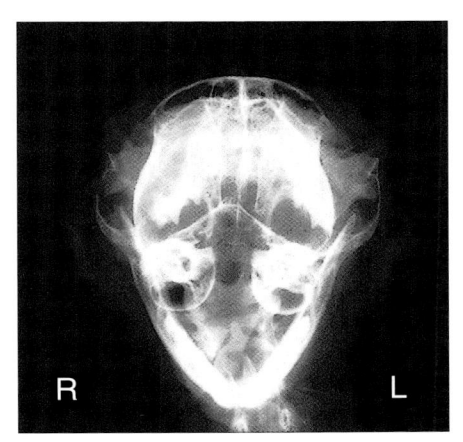

# 3–5: Answers

**3** Strict cage rest is the most important aspect. The patient must rest in a confined space for at least two weeks; it should only be removed to allow it to urinate and defecate. Use of anti-inflammatory medications can be helpful, although they should be withheld during the initial period to encourage rest. The major long-term problem is that over one-third of dogs will suffer a recurrence. Also, the dog could deteriorate during treatment. Physiotherapy must also be delayed until the latter part of the treatment period; recovery of the neurological deficits may be slow and incomplete. It is important that the bladder is regularly emptied of all urine. Urinary retention is the most common cause of postoperative problems in thoracolumbar disc disease. Pharmacological management of urination should be considered whenever urinary function is impaired – see **Q82** and **A82**.

Paraplegic animals are susceptible to the development of decubitus ulcers. Close attention to cleanliness and bedding helps to avoid this problem. Gastrointestinal problems are seen in animals with disc disease; one major risk factor is the use of dexamethasone. Bleeding into the gastrointestinal tract, presenting as 'coffee ground' vomit or melena, should be treated aggressively because of the potentially high mortality rate. Acute pancreatitis may also occur.

**Reference**
Wheeler SJ, Sharp NJH. *Small Animal Spinal Disorders*. London: Mosby-Wolfe, 1994: 107, 203–219.

**4** The C4 vertebra is altered in shape – the ventral margin is disrupted, as is the architecture of the floor of the vertebral canal. The ventral myelogram column is compressed by an extradural lesion over the vertebral body of C4. Little contrast medium has passed cranial to the lesion. The interpretation of the image is of an extradural spinal cord compression in C4 related to a lesion in the vertebral body. This lesion is disturbing the structure of the vertebra, such that there may be a 'pathological' fracture.

The transverse CT image shows loss of bone in the vertebral body, replaced by soft tissue, which is extending into the vertebral canal. Again, the ventral myelogram column is obliterated.

The most likely diagnosis is neoplasia. Differential diagnoses include any tumour of bone origin, ie. osteosarcoma, fibrosarcoma, haemangiosarcoma, chondrosarcoma, myeloma, or a metastatic tumour.

The histopathological diagnosis was osteosarcoma.

**5** There is sclerosis of the left tympanic bulla and increased opacity of the normally air-filled cavity of the tympanic bulla and left external ear canal. Otitis media and nasopharyngeal polyp are the two primary differential diagnoses.

# 6 & 7: Questions

6   While the cat in **Q5** is anaesthetised for radiography, you examine the pharynx and see a pale, tan, fibrous mass. What is the diagnosis and treatment?

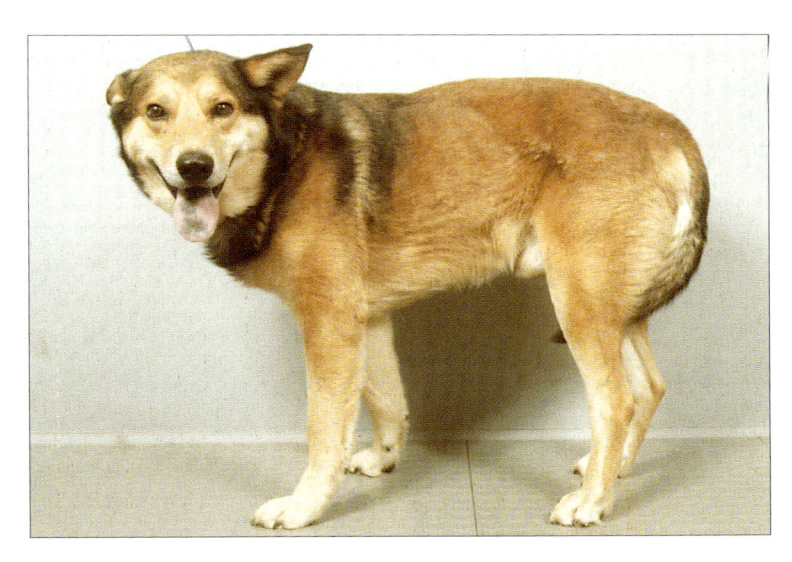

7   A middle-aged, cross-bred dog is presented with a stilted pelvic limb gait and marked pain over the caudal thoracic region (**above**). The rectal temperature is elevated (39.7°C/103.5°F), and the haemogram reveals a leukocytosis with left shift. The dog urinates frequently and urinalysis indicates a purulent cystitis. Thoracic radiographs taken of the conscious dog reveal bone lysis in the T9 and T10 vertebral endplates adjacent to the intervertebral space.
i.   What is the most likely diagnosis?
ii.  What further diagnostic tests would you perform?

# 6 & 7: Answers

**6** This is a nasopharyngeal polyp, a benign fibrous polypoid mass that arises from the middle ear and extends into the nasopharynx or external ear canal. Bacterial infection of the middle ear is common in cats with polyps, but whether infection initiates the development of polyps or is a secondary process is not known. Clinical signs of nasopharyngeal polyps indicate involvement of the upper respiratory system (sneezing, nasal discharge, and stertorous breathing) or middle/inner ear (vestibular dysfunction and Horner's syndrome). Although these masses can often be removed by traction on the pharyngeal portion of the mass, recurrence of the polyp is common with this procedure. Definitive treatment consists of bulla osteotomy with transection of the attachment of the polyp in the tympanic cavity. Horner's syndrome is the most common postoperative complication, but is usually transient. Vestibular dysfunction and facial paralysis can also occur. Complete excision carries a good prognosis, although any preoperative neurological signs may be permanent.

### References
Faulkner JE, Budsberg SC. Results of ventral bulla osteotomy for treatment of middle ear polyps in cats. *J Am Anim Hosp Assn* 1990; **26:** 496–499.
Kapatkin AS, Matthiesen DT, Noone KE *et al*. Results of surgery and long-term follow-up in 31 cats with nasopharyngeal polyps. *J Am Anim Hosp Assn* 1990; **26:** 387–392.
Trevor PB, Martin RA. Tympanic bulla osteotomy for treatment of middle ear disease in cats: 19 cases (1984–1991). *J Am Vet Med Assn* 1993; **202:** 123–128.

**7** i. Discospondylitis.
ii. Blood and urine culture. *Brucella canis* antibody titre in regions where the disease is endemic.

## 8–10: Questions

8   In the dog discussed in Q7, what organisms are most frequently isolated?

9   Congenital diseases of young dogs: link the following breeds, diseases and clinical signs.

| Breed | Disease | Clinical signs |
|---|---|---|
| English springer spaniel | Hypomyelination | Ataxia, hypermetria, proprioceptive deficits, head tremor, visual and menace deficits from 4–9 months |
| Boxer | Fucosidosis | Ataxia, weakness, absent patellar reflexes from 2 months |
| Golden retriever | Cerebellar degeneration and hydrocephalus | Tremor and dysmetria from 3–4 weeks; later improvement to 1 year |
| Weimaraner | Progressive axonopathy | Poor growth, weakness, stilted, shuffling gait, muscle atrophy from 2–6 months |
| Bull mastiff | Muscular dystrophy | Ataxia, hypermetria, proprioceptive deficits at 12–18 months. Progressive to more generalised severe CNS dysfunction |

10   In dogs, the menace response is normally:
a) Present at birth.
b) Developed by 12 weeks.
c) Developed by one year.

## 8–10: Answers

**8** *Staphylococcus intermedius* is by far the most common causative organism, with *Brucella canis*, *Streptococcus* spp. and *Escherichia coli* also found.

**Reference**
Kornegay JN. Discospondylitis. In: Kirk RW (ed). *Current Veterinary Therapy IX*. Philadelphia: Saunders, 1986: 810–814.

**9** See chart below for answers.

| Breed | Disease | Clinical signs |
| --- | --- | --- |
| Weimaraner | Hypomyelination | Tremor and dysmetria from 3–4 weeks; later improvement to 1 year |
| English springer spaniel | Fucosidosis | Ataxia, hypermetria, proprioceptive deficits at 12–18 months. Progressive to more generalised severe CNS dysfunction |
| Bull mastiff | Cerebellar degeneration and hydrocephalus | Ataxia, hypermetria, proprioceptive deficits, head tremor, visual and menace deficits from 4–9 months |
| Boxer | Progressive axonopathy | Ataxia, weakness, absent patellar reflexes from 2 months |
| Golden retriever | Muscular dystrophy | Poor growth, weakness, stilted, shuffling gait, muscle atrophy from 2–6 months |

**10** b) The menace response is absent or slow in puppies up until 12 weeks. Some authors suggest that it may be present at 3–4 weeks of age.

**References**
DeLahunta A. *Veterinary Neuroanatomy and Clinical Neurology*, 2nd edn. Philadelphia: Saunders, 1983: 289.
Oliver JE, Hoerlein BF, Mayhew IG. *Veterinary Neurology*. Philadelphia: Saunders, 1987: 32.
Shores A. Neurologic examination of the canine neonate. *Comp Cont Ed Pract Vet* 1983; 5: 1033–1041.

## 11-13: Questions

**11** What is the use for this material? Are there any potential side-effects of its use?

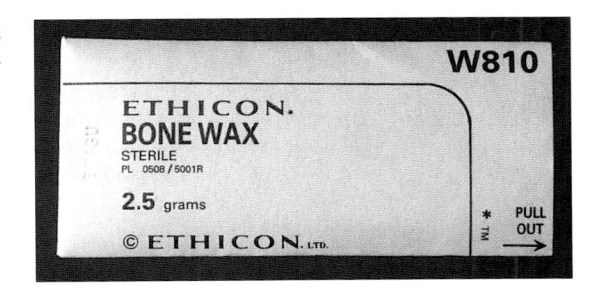

**12** This is a myelogram image of a middle-aged, mixed-breed dog with asymmetrical paraparesis and thoracic spinal pain.
i. Describe the radiographic findings. What do these findings suggest about the location of the lesion relative to the neural structures?
ii. What is the differential diagnosis for such a lesion?
iii. How would you take the case further? What is the prognosis?

**13** This radiograph is of a seven-year-old Lahsa Apso. Neurological abnormalities were restricted to non-ambulatory paraparesis with hyperreflexic patellar reflexes, intact withdrawal reflexes, and lumbar spinal pain. The condition had progressed over five days.
i. What is the localisation of the lesion?
ii. Based on the history and neurological findings, give a realistic differential diagnosis.
iii. What diagnosis is supported by the radiographs?
iv. What laboratory findings would you expect?
v. How could you confirm the diagnosis?
vi. How could you treat the dog and what is the prognosis?

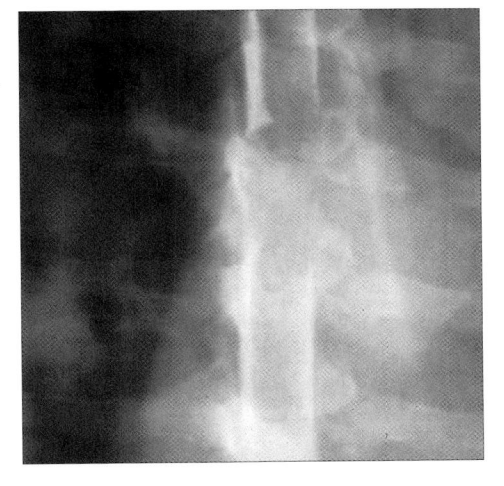

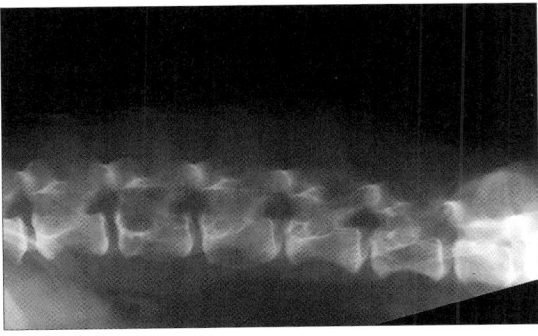

13

## 11–13: Answers

**11** Bone wax is used for haemostasis; it is used to plug small vessels in bone by pressing over the bleeding site. There is a risk of embolisation of this material.

**12 i.** This is a ventrodorsal (or possibly dorsoventral) myelogram in the midthoracic region. There is loss of the contrast columns on the dog's left (**right of the illustration**) and on the right. On the right side, the column spreads in a 'golf-tee' pattern. This suggests an intradural-extramedullary lesion.
**ii.** This is most likely to be a neoplasm. The most common causes are nerve sheath tumour (neurofibrosarcoma, Schwannoma) or meningioma. Other less likely causes would be neuroepithelioma, lymphoma or metastatic lesions.
**iii.** Surgical exploration. It would be wise to screen the dog first for other evidence of neoplasia. At a minimum, chest and abdominal radiographs should be taken.
The prognosis for spinal meningiomas is reasonably good. The neurological status may deteriorate following surgery, but this should improve and many dogs experience lengthy remission. In contrast, nerve sheath tumours have a high rate of local recurrence, even if adjunctive therapy such as radiation is used.

**13 i.** T3–L3 spinal cord – upper motor neuron (UMN) signs in the pelvic limbs, normal thoracic limbs.
**ii.** Disc extrusion.
Neoplasia.
Discospondylitis (less likely in a small breed).
Meningomyelitis – various causes, including canine distemper and granulomatous meningoencephalomyelitis (GME).
Trauma – no compatible history.
**iii.** Multiple radiolucent lesions affecting three vertebrae suggest multifocal neoplasia. Myeloma would be most likely.
**iv.** Hypergammaglobulinaemia and Bence-Jones proteinuria are seen in some cases of myeloma.
**v.** Compatible laboratory findings. Biopsy, possible by fluoroscopic-guided fine-needle aspirate of the lesions.
**vi.** Combination chemotherapy (prednisolone, melphalan) and radiation treatment are useful in some cases.

### Reference
Gorman NT. The haemolymphatic system. In: White RAS (ed). *Manual of Small Animal Oncology.* Cheltenham: BSAVA, 1991: 222.

## 14 & 15: Questions

**14** A five-year-old Golden retriever is evaluated for a 24 hour duration of progressive weakness. Neurological examination reveals an alert, non-ambulatory dog. The postural reactions and spinal reflexes are absent in the pelvic limbs (0) and depressed (+1) in the thoracic limbs. Skeletal muscle tone is markedly decreased. Pain perception and cranial nerves are normal.
i.   What is the neuroanatomical diagnosis?
ii.  What are the differential diagnoses?
iii. What immediate treatment would you recommend?
iv.  What potentially life-threatening complication should you monitor for?

**15** This radiograph is of a nine-year-old Cairn terrier with dysphagia and regurgitation.
i.  Evaluate the radiographs.
ii. What differential diagnoses should you consider?

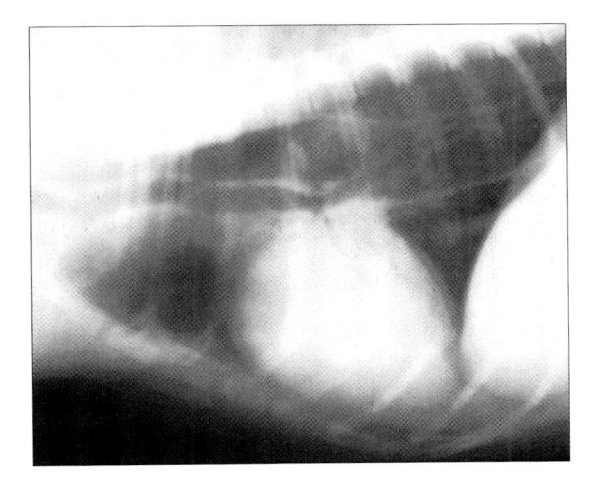

# 14 & 15: Answers

**14 i.** Tetraparesis with decreased or absent spinal cord reflexes indicates diffuse lower motor neuron disease, most likely with involvement of ventral nerve roots, peripheral nerves, or myoneural junctions.
**ii.** Causes of acute progressive signs of diffuse lower motor disease in the dog include polyradiculoneuritis (Coonhound paralysis), tick paralysis, botulism, distal denervating disease, organophosphate intoxication, and coral snake envenomation.
**iii.** The dog should be examined for ticks and any ticks found should be removed. The dog should be dipped for ticks, even if none are found. Improvement within 24 hours of treatment is essentially diagnostic of tick paralysis. If signs do not resolve, polyradiculoneuritis, botulism, or, in certain geographic regions, coral snake envenomation and distal denervating disease, should be considered. These disorders are difficult to confirm unless the history indicates exposure to raccoons, coral snakes, or sources of *Clostridium botulinum*. In any event, treatment for these diseases is largely supportive and dogs will usually recover unless respiratory paralysis develops.
**iv.** Any severely tetraparetic dog should be monitored for respiratory insufficiency. Mechanical ventilation may be necessary if respiratory distress occurs. When available, blood gas determinations are helpful in assessing respiratory function.

**15 i.** The thoracic portion of the oesophagus is enlarged and filled with air. There is a mild increase in opacity of the cranial lung lobe(s). The radiographic diagnosis is megaoesophagus with possible aspiration pneumonia.
**ii.** Reported causes of megaoesophagus in the dog include neuromuscular disorders (myasthenia gravis [MG], polymyositis, polyneuritis), toxins (lead, anticholinesterase), endocrinopathies (hypoadrenocorticism, hypothyroidism), central nervous system lesions, and oesophageal obstruction (stricture, neoplasia, vascular ring anomalies). Most of these disorders can be evaluated by obtaining a thorough history and performing a physical and neurological examination in conjunction with appropriate laboratory evaluation. Approximately 26–37% of dogs with megaoesophagus have acquired MG.

### References
Shelton GD, Willard MD, Cardinet GH, Lindstrom J. Acquired myasthenia gravis: selective involvement of esophageal, pharyngeal, and facial muscles. *J Am Vet Med Assn* 1990; 4: 281–284.
Shelton GD. Megaesophagus secondary to acquired myasthenia gravis. In: Kirk RW, Bonagura JD (eds). *Current Veterinary Therapy XI*. Philadelphia: Saunders, 1994; 581–583.

## 16–18: Questions

**16** Evaluation of serum from the dog in Q15 reveals the presence of antibodies to acetylcholine receptors (AChR), as detected by radioimmunoassay. What is the diagnosis and treatment?

**17** What is wrong with this puppy? What is the underlying abnormality?

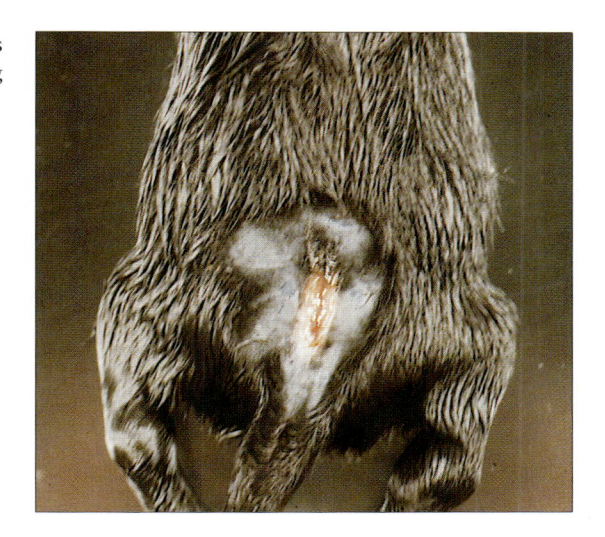

**18** You are presented with a seven-year-old Cavalier King Charles spaniel. The dog had recently been depressed and experiencing seizures. Over the last 24 hours it had developed a head tilt and was unable to walk. Neurological examination revealed a depressed, recumbent dog. The head could be raised at times, when it showed a right head tilt. There were postural reaction deficits in all limbs. There was marked cervical and thoracolumbar pain.
i. What is the lesion localisation?
ii. What are the most likely differential diagnoses based on this localisation?
iii. What further tests would you perform?

## 16–18: Answers

**16** Detection of antibodies to AChR is diagnostic of acquired MG. This autoimmune disease results in destruction of nicotinic acetylcholine receptors at neuromuscular junctions. The classical clinical sign is weakness induced by exercise, but selective involvement of oesophageal, pharyngeal, and facial muscles also occurs. Treatment consists of administration of anticholinesterase drugs. Drugs that inhibit acetylcholinesterase allow acetylcholine that is released from the nerve to interact repeatedly with the limited number of AChRs, resulting in increased force of contraction of muscles. Pyridostigmine (0.5–1 mg/kg, every eight hours) may be administered if oral medication can be tolerated. If severe regurgitation precludes oral medication, neostigmine (0.04–0.05 mg/kg, every six hours) can be administered intramuscularly. The dosage may need to be adjusted based on the individual animal's response. Immunosuppressive dosages of glucocorticoids are recommended when weakness is not adequately controlled by anticholinesterase drugs.

To decrease regurgitation, the dog should be fed and watered in an upright position. To provide nutrition and decrease the likelihood of aspiration, a gastrotomy tube should be placed in dogs with severe regurgitation. Antibiotics are indicated in animals with pneumonia, although aminoglycosides may exacerbate muscle weakness in dogs with myasthenia gravis.

Medical treatment should continue until the serum AchR antibody titre is normal. Many dogs will undergo spontaneous remission. The presence of severe aspiration pneumonia or pharyngeal weakness indicates a more guarded prognosis.

### References
Shelton GD, Willard MD, Cardinet GH, Lindstrom J. Acquired myasthenia gravis: selective involvement of esophageal, pharyngeal, and facial muscles. *J Am Vet Med Assn* 1990; 4: 281–284.
Shelton GD. Megaesophagus secondary to acquired myasthenia gravis. In: Kirk RW, Bonagura JD (eds). *Current Veterinary Therapy XI*. Philadelphia: Saunders, 1994; 581–583.
Hopkins AL. Canine myasthenia gravis. *J Small Anim Pract*1992; 33: 477–484.


**17** Spina bifida. In this patient there is exposure of the underlying neural tissue. There is a failure of fusion of the dorsal elements of the neural tube in the embryo, leading to abnormalities of the vertebra and spinal cord.


**18** i. Multifocal.
   Seizures = forebrain.
   Head tilt and postural reaction deficits = central vestibular/brainstem.
   Cervical pain = cervical.
   Thoracolumbar pain = thoracolumbar.
ii. Most multifocal disorders in dogs are inflammatory, although occasionally they are neoplastic.
iii. Cerebrospinal fluid (CSF) analysis; serology.

# 25 & 26: Questions

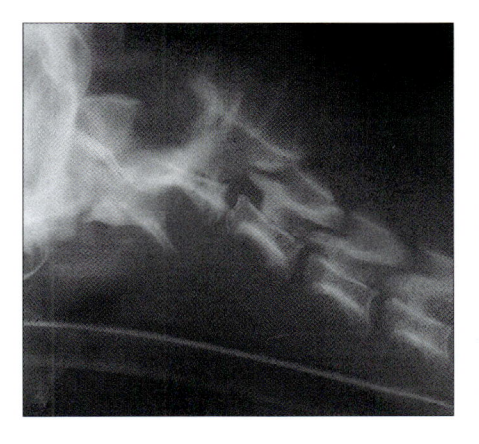

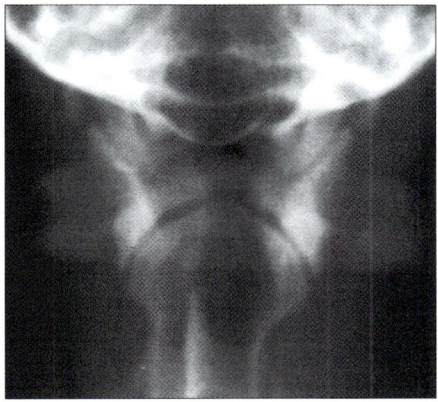

25  The radiographs (**above**) are of the dog described in **Q24**
i.   Describe the radiographic findings.
ii.  What are the pathological changes that may underlie this condition?
iii. How may the condition be treated?
iv.  What is the prognosis?

26  A three-year-old Pointer presents with a two month duration of weight loss and lethargy. Rectal temperature is 39.5º C (103.3ºF). Marked signs of pain are elicited on palpation of the cranial lumbar vertebrae. The gait is stiff in the pelvic limbs but there are no other neurological deficits. What are your diagnostic considerations?

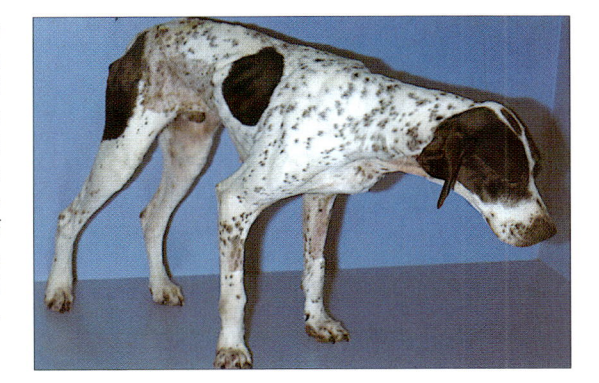

## 25 & 26: Answers

**25 i.** The lateral radiograph shows an abnormal widening between the dorsal arch of C1 and the spinous process of C2. The alignment of the vertebral canal between these vertebrae is disrupted. The ventrodorsal film shows absence of the dens.

**ii.** Absent or small dens.

Fracture or separation of the dens.

Damage to or insufficiency of the transverse ligament of the atlas.

**iii.** Non-surgical treatment – cage rest and splinting.

Surgical treatment – dorsal wiring (not recommended) or ventral lag screws and bone graft. Radiograph on right was taken postoperatively following lag screw fixation.

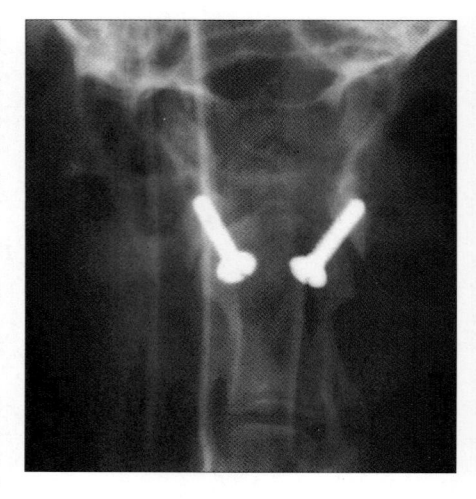

**iv.** The prognosis is variable, mainly depending on the original neurological status; the more severe the deficits, the less favourable the outlook. Dogs with neck pain and mild deficits have a good prognosis. Dogs with tetraplegia have a guarded outlook.

**26** Primary considerations are discospondylitis, vertebral osteomyelitis, focal meningitis, and neoplasia. Trauma and intervertebral disc extrusion can also cause spinal pain but are less likely considering the systemic signs of fever and lethargy.

# 27–29: Questions

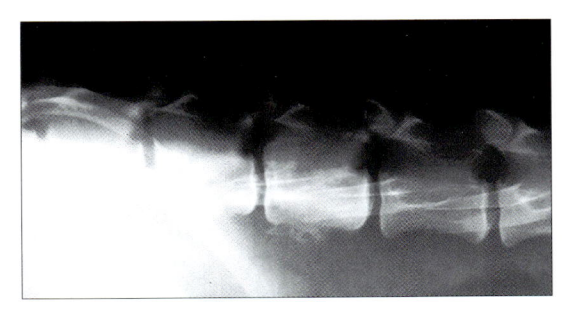

**27** Evaluate the radiographs (**above** and **right**) of the lumbar spine of the dog in **Q26**.

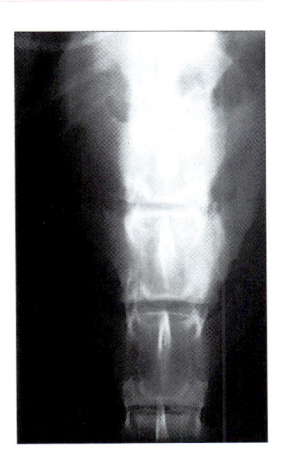

**28** A three-year-old Cocker spaniel is presented for evaluation of seizures. Examination reveals a depressed, ataxic dog with a head tilt to the right. The rectal temperature is 39.6°C (103.4°F). Postural reactions are decreased on the right (+1). Chest radiographs are taken because of increased lung sounds. Interpret the results of the neurological examination and radiographs.

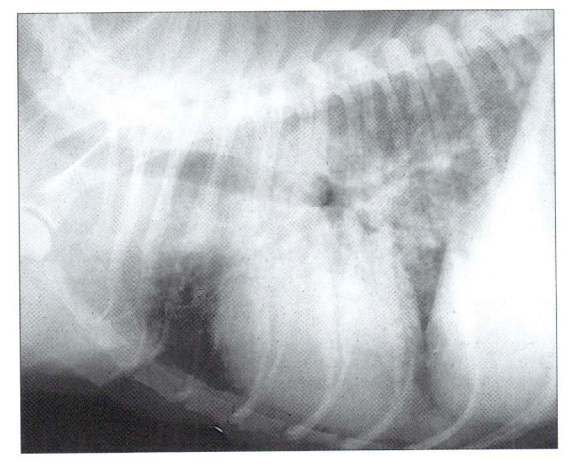

**29** Cerebrospinal fluid from the dog in **Q28** has a protein concentration of 107 mg/dl and 57 nucleated cells per µl. The cytology preparation is shown. What is the diagnosis and treatment?

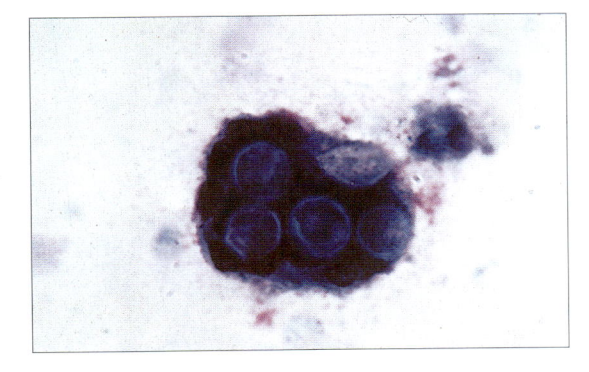

## 27–29: Answers

**27** There is a proliferative lesion involving the L1–L3 vertebral bodies and the lamina of L3. These changes are consistent with spondylitis, especially due to migrating plant material. Aspiration of paravertebral soft tissue showed a mixed infection, including *Actinomyces*. Treatment of spondylitis caused by *Actinomyces* includes surgical drainage and antibiotic administration.

**28** Seizures indicate forebrain disease. The right head tilt and hemiparesis indicate a lesion involving the right side of the brainstem. Thus, this dog has multifocal lesions. The thoracic radiographs show a diffuse, nodular interstitial pattern. Systemic mycoses, such as histoplasmosis and blastomycosis, should be considered.

**29** There are several organisms with a central basophilic nucleus and an outer clear capsule, consistent with the appearance of *Blastomyces dermatitidis*.

The traditional treatment of meningoencephalitis due to *Blastomyces* infection has been administration of amphotericin B (0.5 mg/kg diluted in 5% dextrose via slow intravenous infusion). Treatment should be given every other day unless there is laboratory evidence of renal damage, such as a serum urea nitrogen concentration greater than 50 mg/dl. A cumulative dose of 8–10 mg/kg is required to cure blastomycosis. Itraconazole (5 mg/kg/day, orally) may be as effective as amphotericin B in dogs with blastomycosis. Treatment should be continued until all clinical signs have been resolved for 30 days.

Although about 80% of dogs with blastomycosis can be effectively treated, the prognosis is more guarded in cases of central nervous system involvement. Approximately 20% of dogs will have a relapse, necessitating re-treatment.

### References
Terrell CL, Hughes CE. Antifungal agents used for deep-seated mycotic infections. *Mayo Clin Proc* 1992; 67: 69–91.
Legendre A. Blastomycosis. In: Greene CE (ed). *Infectious Diseases of the Dog and Cat*. Philadelphia: Saunders, 1990: 669–678.

# 30 & 31: Questions

**30** Head injuries may cause acute brainstem lesions, or progressive forebrain lesions with secondary brain herniation. How do these situations differ?

**31** These radiographs are of a five-month-old Yorkshire terrier with progressive stiffness and tetraparesis over six weeks.
i. What is the diagnosis?
ii. What is the treatment and prognosis?

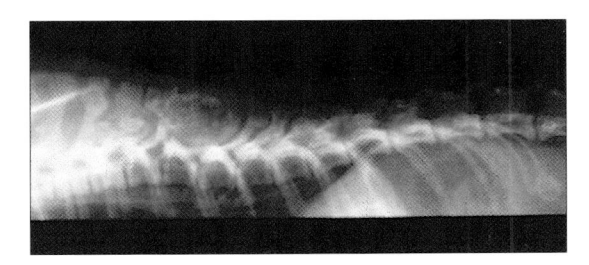

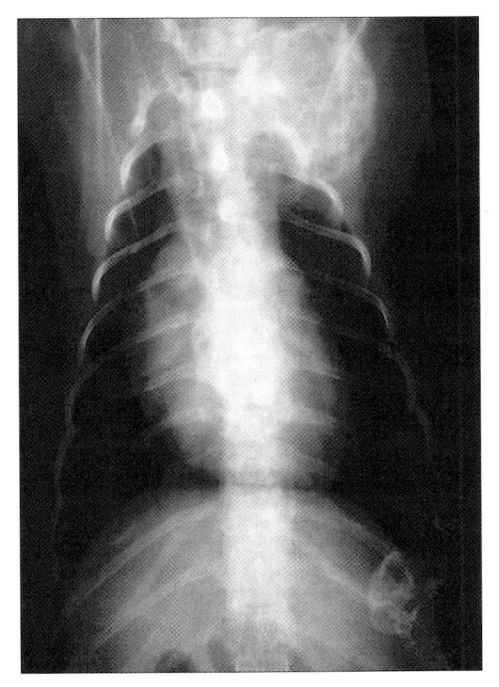

# 30 & 31: Answers

|  | Brainstem | Forebrain |
|---|---|---|
| Onset | Acute, early | Delayed |
| Course | Usually non-progressive after initial severe presentation | Progressive |
| Level of consciousness | Stupor or coma | Depressed, progressing by stages to coma |
| Locomotor status | Decerebrate rigidity or paralysis | Weakness progressing to severe paresis and eventual decerebrate rigidity |
| Pupils | Constricted early, later dilated | Early responsive, later sluggish pupillary reflexes, becoming fixed dilated |

30  See chart above.

### Reference
Griffiths IR. Central nervous system trauma. In: Oliver JE, Hoerlein BF, Mayhew IG (eds). *Veterinary Neurology*. Philadelphia: Saunders, 1987: 303–320.


31  i. There are multiple, cystic expansile lesions involving the left first and tenth ribs, and the T2–T10 vertebrae. These findings are consistent with multiple cartilagenous exostoses, a benign proliferative lesion of the epiphyseal region. Any bone formed by endochondral ossification may be affected, with the vertebrae, ribs, and long bones being the most frequent sites. Myelography is necessary to identify the specific site of spinal cord compression.
ii. Surgical excision is recommended for cartilagenous exostoses causing neurological dysfunction. The prognosis for recovery is good for mature animals. Multiple operations may be required in immature animals as lesions may continue to grow until normal bone growth at the epiphysis stops.

### References
Prata RG, Stoll SG, Zaki FA. Spinal cord compression caused by osteocartilagenous exostoses of the spine in two dogs. *J Am Vet Med Assn* 1975; **166**: 371–375.
Gambardella PC, Osborne CA, Stevens JB. Multiple cartilagenous exostoses in the dog. *J Am Vet Med Assn* 1975; **166**: 761–768.

## 32 & 33: Questions

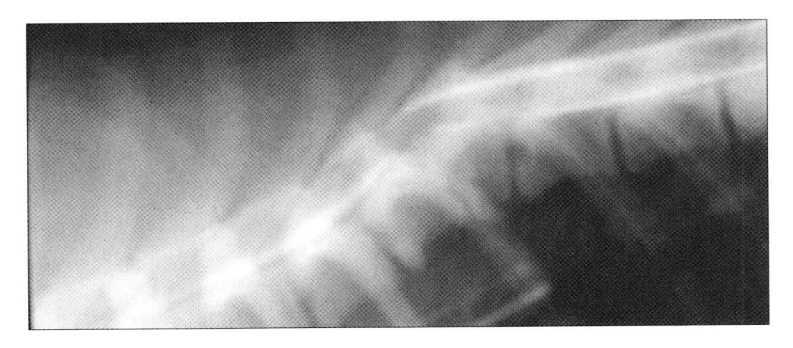

**32** The myelogram (**above**) is of a nine-month-old terrier cross that has always had difficulty using the pelvic limbs. When supported, the dog is able to walk, although the gait is very ataxic, with little coordination between the thoracic and pelvic limbs. Patellar reflexes are exaggerated with clonus, and the flexor reflex is intact, with a crossed extensor. Deep pain perception is absent in the pelvic limbs. Interpret the results of the neurological examination and radiographs.

**33** Signalment: 10-month-old male Pug.
History: seizures of two days duration.
Clinical findings: dull, depressed, twitching facial muscles. Severely tetraparetic, worse on right. No postural reactions on right; no menace response on right, but pupillary light reflexes and palpebral reflex intact. Reduced facial sensation on right. Cervical and thoracolumbar spinal pain.
i.  Localise the lesion.
ii. Give a differential diagnosis.
iii. What tests would you consider? Are there any hazards in these?

## 32 & 33: Answers

**32** Neurological examination indicates a lesion of the T3–L3 spinal cord segments. The lack of deep pain perception in a dog that is able to walk usually indicates that the dog is spinal walking. Pattern generators located in the spinal cord can induce stepping movements independent of input from the brain. Animals with transection of the thoracolumbar portion of the spinal cord will occasionally develop the ability to generate the basic movements of the step cycle in the pelvic limbs. When the thoracic limbs start walking, the pelvic limb movements can be adequate to support the animal during locomotion, a process called spinal walking or spinal stepping.

The myelogram shows a dorsal hemivertebrae of one of the mid-thoracic vertebrae with associated spinal cord compression. Hemivertebrae is a developmental anomaly that is due to failure of ossification of the ventral half of the vertebral body. Although this is often an incidental finding, in severe cases such as this, narrowing of the vertebral canal can cause compression of the spinal cord. Surgical decompression and stabilisation of the affected vertebrae may be successful in some cases. The chronic course and absence of deep pain perception in this dog indicates that the spinal cord injury is probably irreversible.

**References**
Grillner S. Locomotion in vertebrates: central mechanisms and reflex interaction. *Physiolog Revs* 1975; **55**: 247–302.
Bailey CS. An embryological approach to the clinical significance of congenital vertebral and spinal cord abnormalities. *J Am Anim Hosp Assn* 1975; **11**: 426–434.

**33** i. Multifocal: seizures, absent menace response with intact pupillary light reflex and palpebral reflex = forebrain; severe asymmetrical tetraparesis = cervical spine or brainstem; cervical pain = cervical spine; thoracolumbar pain = thoracolumbar spine.
ii. Inflammatory CNS disease or neoplasia.
iii. Intracranial imaging – CT or magnetic resonance imaging (MRI) and CSF collection. Both tests require general anaesthesia, which can increase intracranial pressure and contribute to brain herniation, particularly if the animal becomes hypoxic or inhalation anaesthetics (especially halothane) are used (see **A87**). Collection of CSF can also lead to brain herniation by reducing CSF pressure caudal to the foramen magnum relative to that cranial to the foramen magnum.

## 34–36: Questions

**34** In the dog described in Q33, all the laboratory results are unremarkable, apart from some evidence of dehydration. The CSF findings are as follows:
WBC – 143 per µl; all mononuclear cells, mixture of lymphocytes and macrophages. Protein – 33 mg/dl.
i. What could the diagnosis be?
ii. What is the prognosis?

**35** Localise the lesion in the following patient: the right pupil is dilated and only the left pupil constricts when light is shone into either eye.

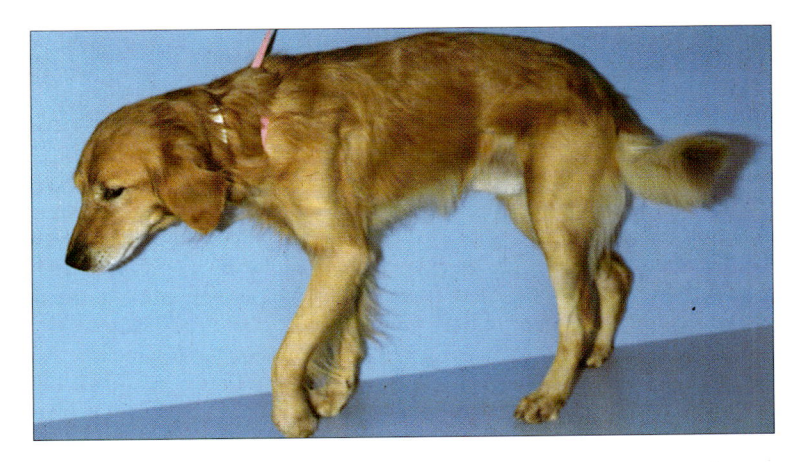

**36** A six-year-old Golden retriever (**above**) is evaluated for left thoracic limb lameness of six months' duration. Initially there was a subtle lameness of the affected limb. No cause for the lameness was detected despite multiple radiographs and arthrocentesis. Two months before presentation the dog began dragging the limb. There is atrophy of the limb and a weak flexor reflex. The cutaneous trunci (panniculus) reflex is absent on the left. Pain is elicited on palpation of the left axilla. No other neurological deficits are detected. What is your tentative diagnosis and recommendation?

## 34–36: Answers

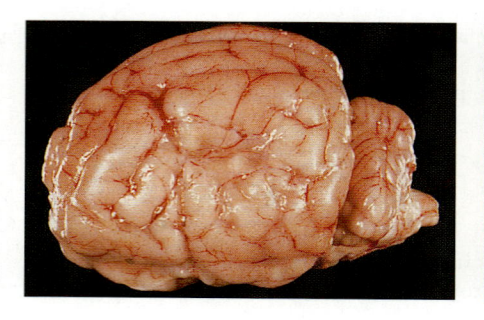

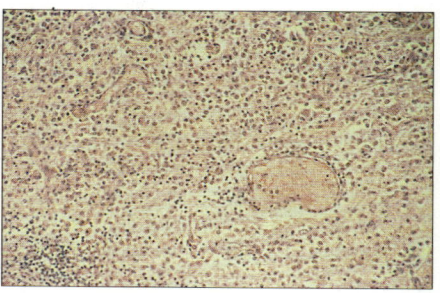

**34 i.** Pug encephalitis, GME. Gross pathology and histolopathology sections of pug encephalitis are shown (**above**).
**ii.** Some cases of GME can be managed for periods with immunosuppressive doses of corticosteroids. However, the long-term outlook for both diseases is poor.

**35** Right pupil or parasympathetic portion of the right oculomotor nerve (cranial nerve III). To test the ability of the pupil to constrict, 2% pilocarpine (a direct-acting parasympathomimetic) is instilled into each eye. If the affected pupil remains dilated and the other pupil constricts, iris disease or prior application of a mydriatic drug is likely. If the affected pupil constricts sooner than the other pupil, a postganglionic lesion of the oculomotor nerve (ciliary ganglion or short ciliary nerves) is present, causing denervation supersensitivity. A preganglionic lesion (parasympathetic nucleus of cranial nerve III or oculomotor nerve) can be evaluated by instilling 0.5% physostigmine (an indirect-acting parasympathomimetic) into each eye. If the affected pupil constricts before the other pupil, a preganglionic lesion is present. If there is a postganglionic lesion, the affected pupil will not constrict.

### Reference
Neer TM, Carter JD. Anisocoria in dogs and cats: ocular and neurological causes. *Compend Contin Educat Pract Vet* 1987; 8: 817–823.

**36** Left brachial plexus neoplasia, most likely a nerve sheath tumor. There is a chronic, progressive lesion involving multiple nerves of the left brachial plexus, including the lateral thoracic nerve (leading to absent cutaneous trunci reflex). Definitive diagnosis requires surgical exploration of the brachial plexus. Myelography should be performed to exclude compression of the spinal cord due to proximal extension of the tumour along nerve roots.

## 37–39: Questions

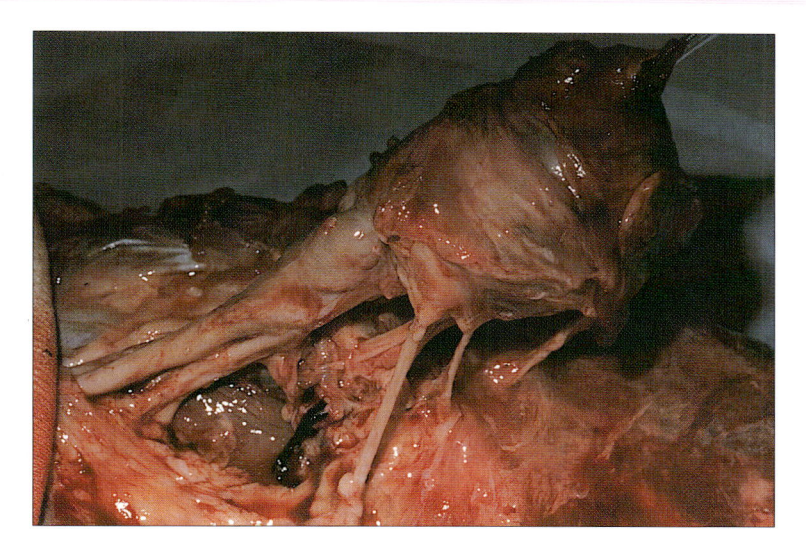

**37** Surgical exploration of the axilla of the dog in **Q36** reveals a large mass involving the brachial plexus. What is the prognosis?

**38** Regarding management of status epilepticus, the preferred route of administration of diazepam is intravenous injection. In cases where an intravenous injection is impossible, diazepam is best administered:
a) Orally.
b) Intramuscularly.
c) Subcutaneously.
d) Per rectum.

**39** A six-year-old Labrador suffers a road traffic accident. Following treatment the dog is discharged from your clinic. The following day, no neurological deficits are seen. One week later the dog is depressed, begins to circle to the right and, over a few hours, starts to drag the left pelvic limb. Neurological examination reveals a depressed dog with a marked tendency to circle to the right and postural reaction deficits on the left side. Also, the dog is blind in the left eye and there is no menace response in that eye, but the pupillary light reflex and palpebral reflex are intact.
i. Localise the lesion.
ii. What may be happening?
iii. What diagnostic tests would you perform?

## 37-39: Answers

**37** These findings are typical of an advanced nerve sheath tumour. Because surgical excision requires division of multiple nerves, amputation of the limb is often necessary. Radiation therapy may be effective is slowing recurrence, but most of these tumours will recur and eventually involve the spinal cord.

### Reference
Targett MP, Dyce J, Houlton JEF. Tumours involving the nerve sheaths of the forelimb in dogs. *J Small Anim Pract* 1993; 34: 221–225.

**38** d) Per rectum. Diazepam is absorbed rapidly following per rectal administration. This route is useful when a peripheral vein is not accessible. Per rectal diazepam (0.5 mg/kg of injectable solution) administered by owners is useful in the management of status epilepticus and clusters of multiple seizures.

### Reference
Podell M. The use of diazepam per rectum at home for the acute management of cluster seizures in dogs. *J Vet Intern Med* 1995; 8: 68–74.

**39** i. Right forebrain. Animals with unilateral forebrain lesions may have contralateral postural reaction deficits and menace response deficits. The intact palpebral reflex indicates that the efferent pathway of the menace response (the facial nerve – cranial nerve VII) is intact. The intact pupillary light reflex localises the menace deficit to the visual pathways, caudal to the level of the lateral geniculate nucleus. Finally, animals with forebrain lesions tend to circle towards the side of the lesion, although this is somewhat variable.
ii. The progressive nature of the disorder suggests that there is a mass effect in the cerebral cortex. This could be due to an expanding lesion, or to the brain's response to the presence of a lesion (mainly oedema), or both. Following trauma, haemorrhage or haematoma formation is likely. If there had been a penetrating injury to the head, abscess formation should also be considered. There could also be a totally coincidental disease process not related to the trauma.
iii. Intracranial imaging (CT or MRI) is the most important test. CSF collection could be performed if the scan is normal. It would not be wise to collect CSF before scanning the dog, as there is a risk of brain herniation in a patient with such a history.

## 40–42: Questions

**40** This is a CT scan of the dog discussed in Q39. Describe and interpret the features.

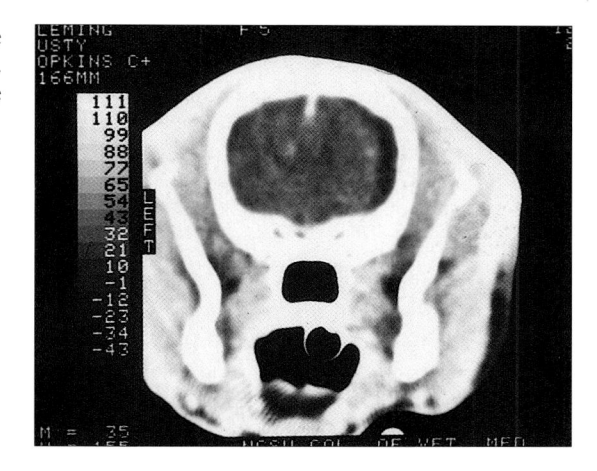

**41** This four-month-old female Labrador has progressively lost pelvic limb function over the past two weeks. It is also urinary and faecally incontinent. The dog is paraplegic with pelvic limb rigidity. Spinal reflexes are absent in the pelvic limbs and there is no anal reflex. The bladder is readily expressed manually. There is diffuse muscle pain in the pelvic limbs. The cranial abdomen is painful and the liver large.
i. Localise the lesion and give a differential diagnosis.
ii. What other tests would you perform?
Laboratory evaluations reveal mild hepatic dysfunction and an eosinophilia （1.4 x $10^3$ per µl; normal = 0.1–0.2 per µl). CSF analysis is normal, as are spinal radiographs. A serum *Toxoplasma gondii* titre was negative; *Neospora caninum* titre was 1/3200 (clinical infection indicated by titres greater than 1/800; subclinical exposure if greater than 1/250).
iii. What is the diagnosis? How would you treat the dog?
iv. What is the prognosis?

**42** i. How are upper motor neuron lesions and lower motor neuron lesions similar?
ii. How are they different?

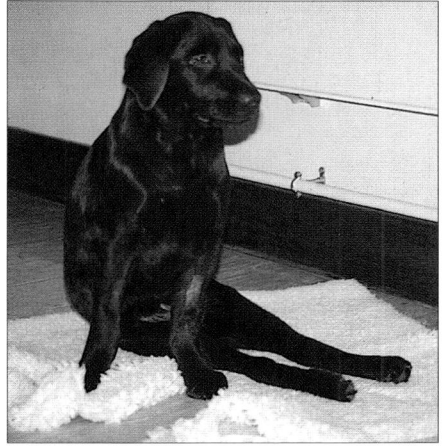

## 40–42: Answers

**40** Within the cranial vault there is an area of tissue that is less dense than the brain parenchyma. This lies under the calvarium on the right side. There is evidence of mass effect – that is, displacement of the falx cerebri to the left and asymmetry of the lateral ventricles. There is no evidence of a large contrast-enhancing lesion. This is probably a subdural haematoma, as was confirmed at surgery.

**Reference**
Hopkins AL, Wheeler SJ. Subdural haematoma in a dog. *Vet Surg* 1991; **20**: 413–417.

**41** i. The neurological lesion can be localised to the L4–S3 spinal cord segments, based on the lower motor neuron (LMN) signs in the pelvic limbs, bladder, and perineum. The muscle pain and rigidity suggests a myopathy, and the hepatomegaly indicates a systemic disease.
ii. Haematology, biochemistry, urinalysis, spinal radiographs, abdominal investigation (radiographs, ultrasound). Later investigations may include CSF analysis, myelography, and *Toxoplasma* and *Neospora* titres.
iii. *Neospora caninum* infection involving liver, nervous system, and muscle. Clindamycin and trimethoprim/suphonamide in combination are recommended.
iv. Guarded – treatment may be more successful if initiated before pelvic limb hyperextension has occurred.

**Reference**
Dubey JP. *Neospora caninum* : a look at a new *Toxoplasma*-like parasite of dogs and other animals. *Compend Contin Educ Pract Vet* 1990; **12**: 653–660.

**42** i. The cell bodies of upper motor neurons (UMNs) are located in the cerebral cortex, basal nuclei, and brainstem nuclei. The axons of the UMNs descend through white matter tracts to synapse on lower motor neurons (LMNs) located in the nuclei of cranial nerves (cranial nerves III–VII, IX–XII) and in the grey matter of the spinal cord. A lesion affecting the UMNs and a lesion affecting the LMNs will both cause decreased or absent voluntary movement, called paresis or paralysis, respectively. The degree of dysfunction depends on the severity of the lesion. Thus, the presence or degree of weakness does not differentiate between an UMN lesion and a LMN lesion.
ii. UMN lesions cause loss of motor function caudal to the lesion. LMN lesions cause loss of function only in muscles innervated by the affected LMNs. UMN lesions are characterised by normal to increased spinal reflexes and muscle tone. A crossed extensor reflex, mass reflex, or extensor toe reflex may be seen, especially with chronic lesions. LMN lesions are characterised by decreased or absent reflexes, muscle flaccidity, and early severe muscle atrophy.

# 43–45: Questions

**43** What neurological deficit is seen in this 11-year-old Jack Russell terrier? The condition is chronic, progressive, and involves only the right side of the head. There is no history of trauma. What is the likely diagnosis?

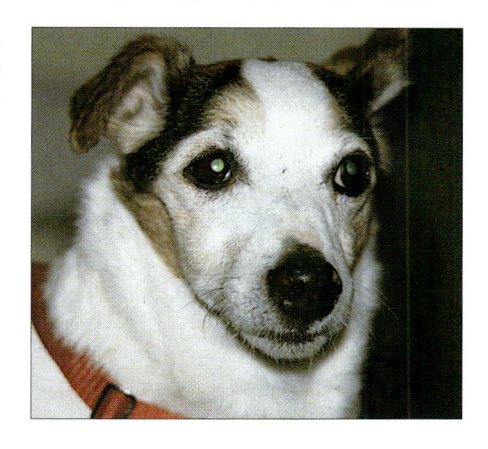

**44** A five-year-old Poodle presents with neck pain. The neurological examination is normal, apart from cervical and thoracolumbar pain. Spinal radiographs reveal widespread disc degeneration, and narrow intervertebral spaces in the cervical and thoracolumbar spine. What tests would you perform to make the diagnosis?

**45** This Cavalier King Charles spaniel is presented with a head tilt.
**i.** What part of the nervous system is involved?
**ii.** What are the major divisions of this system, and how may lesions in the areas be differentiated?

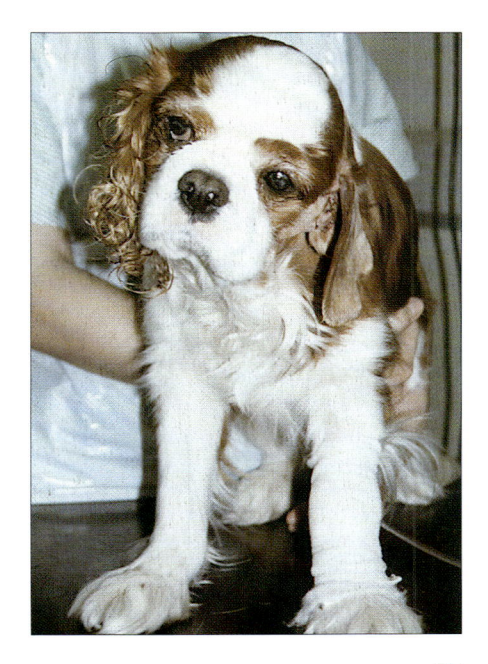

## 43–45: Answers

**43** Severe atrophy of the muscle of mastication: thus motor paralysis of the trigeminal nerve (cranial nerve V). A unilateral lesion is most likely to be due to a neoplasm of the nerve. (See also **Q68**.)

**44** Thorough physical and neurological examinations, haematology, biochemistry, urinalysis, CSF analysis, and myelography.

**45 i.** A head tilt indicates vestibular syndrome – that is, dysfunction of the vestibular system. This dog also has facial paralysis and Horner's syndrome on the left side.

**ii.** The vestibular system comprises the distal receptors in the inner ear, the vestibular nerve (part of cranial nerve VIII), the vestibular nuclei in the brainstem, and parts of the cerebellum. Caudal and rostral projections of the vestibular system influence limb muscles and the extraocular muscles.

The important clinical differentiation is between peripheral (receptor and nerve) and central (brainstem) vestibular disease (see Table).

| Feature | Peripheral | Central |
|---|---|---|
| Head tilt | Yes | Yes |
| Ataxia | Yes | Yes |
| Proprioceptive deficits | No | Ipsilateral |
| Paresis | No | Ipsilateral |
| Nystagmus | Yes† | Yes† |
| Variable nystagmus* | No | Yes |
| Other cranial nerves | VII | Multiple |

* Direction or character of nystagmus changes when head position is altered.
† Nystagmus is generally characterised by its fast phase; that is, when the fast phase is to the right, this is termed a 'right nystagmus'. The direction of the nystagmus is generally away from the lesion. It may be easier to remember that the slow phase of the nystagmus is generally towards the side of the lesion.

## 46–48: Questions

**46** Neurological examination of the dog shown in Q45 reveals normal postural reactions, nystagmus with the fast phase to the right, left facial paralysis, left head tilt, and left Horner's syndrome.
i. Where is the lesion?
ii. What are the possible causes of this type of disorder?
iii. Which is most likely?
iv. How would you pursue the diagnosis?

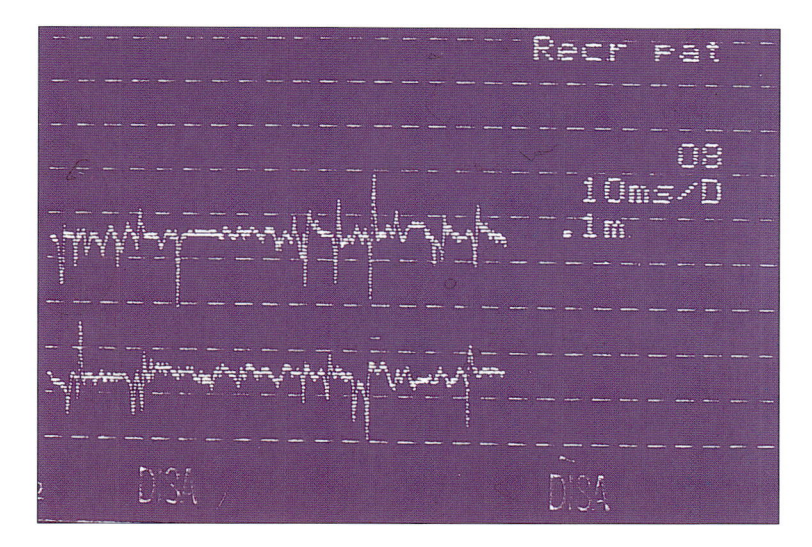

**47** You refer a dog with generalised muscle wasting and weakness for an electromyographic (EMG) examination. The report (which is accompanied by this trace) describes 'diffuse spontaneous electrical activity, comprising fibrillations and positive sharp waves, in all limb muscles'. What does this indicate and what further tests would you perform?

**48** You are preparing to anaesthetise a dog for a CT scan to investigate an intracranial lesion. What potential complications should be anticipated and how would you try to avoid these?

39

## 46–48: Answers

**46 i.** Peripheral vestibular.
**ii.** Neuropathy (possibly hypothyroid-related); congenital; neoplasia; otitis media/interna; iatrogenic (ear swabbing, flushing, or surgery); idiopathic; trauma; toxic - ototoxic drugs.
**iii.** Otitis media/interna.
**iv.** Physical examination. Thorough otic examination under anaesthesia, ensuring that the tympanic membranes are evaluated. Bulla series radiographs. If abnormal and suggesting otitis, collection of middle ear contents for cytology and culture. If normal, check thyroid function. In progressive disease, intracranial imaging (CT, MRI) may be indicated, as peripheral lesions could progress to a central location.

**47** This type of finding on an EMG examination is indicative either of denervation or primary muscle disease. It would be important to know if the motor and sensory nerve conduction studies were normal. Serum biochemistry, particularly creatine kinase (CK) should be evaluated. Elevated CK concentrations are seen in muscle disease rather than in denervation.

**48** General anaesthesia may lead to an increase in intracranial pressure, which could precipitate brain herniation. To avoid this, two techniques are employed:
• The first is by selection of appropriate agents. The pure agonist narcotic analgesics (morphine, oxymorphone) should be avoided, as they lead to increased intra-cranial pressure (ICP). Most inhalation anaesthetics (particularly halothane) increase cerebral blood flow, which can also increase ICP. Isoflurane is the agent with the least tendency to do this. Barbiturates tend to reduce cerebral blood flow and are beneficial in this regard.
• The second important consideration is the ventilation of the animal. Increases in $pCO_2$ increase cerebral blood flow, which tends to increase ICP. Thus, it is important that the airway is maintained. Hyperventilating the patient, to drive down $pCO_2$ to 25–30 mmHg, can have a significant beneficial effect.

Seizure activity on recovery should be avoided, as this can contribute to increased oxygen demand by the brain and cytotoxic brain oedema. An intravenous catheter should be left in place, and suitable medication made available.

If herniation is occurring, hyperventilation is the first course of action. It may be necessary to administer mannitol and frusemide to reduce the brain volume (see **Q84** and **A84**).

### Reference
Shores A. Neuroanesthesia: a review of the effects of anaesthetic agents on cerebral blood flow and intracranial pressure in the dog. *Vet Surg* 1985: **14**: 257–263.

# 49–51: Questions

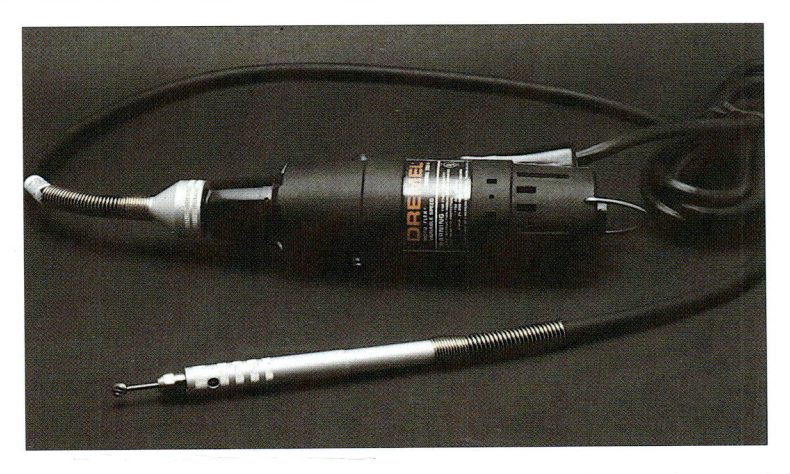

**49** This instrument, the 'Dremel' model drill (**above**), is often used as a substitute for pneumatic equipment in neurosurgery. What are its advantages and disadvantages?

**50** A Dalmatian breeder brings you two puppies, from a litter of eight, which are suspected to be deaf. As far as you can tell, this is the case. How could this be confirmed? What are the implications for the litter and what action would you take?

**51** A six-year-old domestic cat has become progressively ataxic over two weeks. It has also become aggressive and appears to be hyper-responsive to noises and touch. The cat tends to sit crouched in the examination room. It is difficult to examine, but postural reactions, spinal reflexes, and cranial nerve reflexes appear normal, and there is no spinal hyperaesthesia.
i. What conditions would you consider in differential diagnosis?
ii. How would you attempt to confirm the diagnosis?

# 49–51: Answers

**49** This type of drill is considerably less expensive than pneumatic systems and has acceptable performance. Sterilisation is a problem; ethylene oxide systems can be used, but their availability is restricted. Methods of wrapping the instrument in sterile drapes have been suggested but are less satisfactory.

**Reference**
Walker TL, Roberts RE, Kinkaid SA, Bratton GR. The use of electric drills as an alternative to pneumatic equipment in spinal surgery. *J Am Anim Hosp Assn* 1981; **17**: 605–612.

**50** Use of brainstem auditory-evoked potential (BAEP) testing. Click sounds are applied to the ears via headphones and the evoked brain responses are detected via surface electrodes. The technique can determine the level in the auditory pathway of hearing deficits, and can demonstrate unilateral deafness (which is difficult to detect clinically).

Deafness is an hereditary condition in Dalmatians. Some dogs may be unilaterally deaf, and therefore clinically normal, but able to transmit the defect. All puppies in the litter should be tested by BAEP and affected puppies should not be used for breeding. Deaf animals are difficult to manage and many breeders elect to have them euthanased.

**Reference**
Strain GM, Kearney MT, Gignac IJ et al. Brainstem auditory-evoked potential assessment of congenital deafness in Dalmatians: associations with phenotypic markers. *J Vet Intern Med* 1992; **6**: 175–182.

**51 i.** Any intracranial disease affecting the forebrain could be implicated. The main considerations are:
Feline spongiform encephalopathy.
Neoplasia – usually meningioma.
Meningoencephalitis, possibly related to feline infectious peritonitis (FIP).
**ii.** Intracranial imaging and CSF analysis. Any cat with ill-defined neurological signs warrants serological evaluation for feline leukaemia virus (FeLV) and feline immunodeficiency virus (FIV).

## 52–54: Questions

**52** In the cat described in Q51, the laboratory evaluations, serology, CT scan, and CSF analysis are normal. What is the most likely diagnosis? How could this be confirmed and what are the implications?

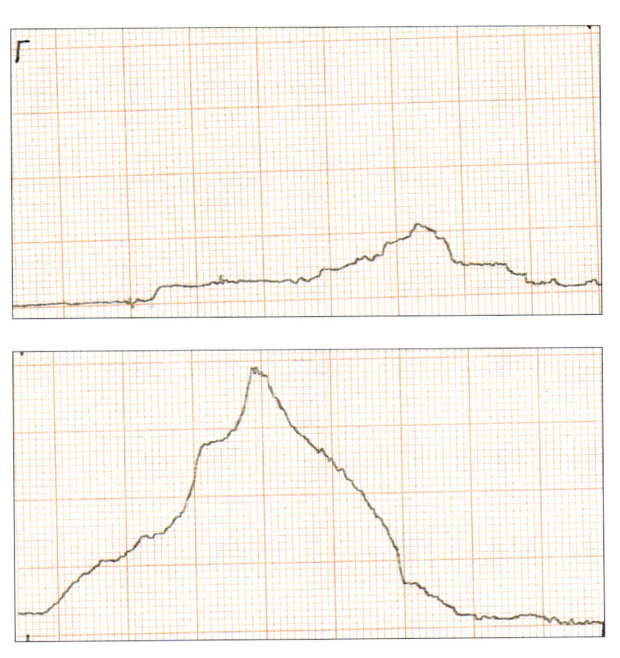

**53** A seven-year-old, spayed, female Bull mastiff has a six-month duration of urinary incontinence. The owner reports the dog often dribbles urine, especially during the night or when it is active. The owner feels that the dog's water consumption and frequency of urination are normal. No neurological deficits are detected; the perineal reflex is normal. The dog urinates normally when taken outside, after which the bladder cannot be palpated. Results of urinalysis are normal with a specific gravity of 1.031. The dog is referred for diagnostic evaluation. A urethral pressure profile reveals the maximum urethral pressure is decreased (**top**). For comparison, a normal urethral pressure profile from a female dog is shown (**bottom**). A cystometrogram is normal. What is the diagnosis and treatment?

**54** What are four indications for therapeutic drug monitoring of serum phenobarbitone concentrations?

## 52–54: Answers

**52** Feline spongiform encephalopathy. This disease carries a hopeless prognosis. Confirmation of the diagnosis is by histopathological examination. The disease is notifiable to the Ministry of Agriculture in the UK if there is reasonable suspicion of it being present on laboratory or pathological evaluations.

**53** Dribbling of urine in an animal that voluntarily urinates suggests urethral incompetence. This was confirmed by finding decreased urethral pressure. The lack of other neurological deficits indicates that a primary defect involving the urethral sphincters is most likely. The most common cause of decreased sphincter tone with a normal detrusor reflex is primary sphincter incompetence. Oestrogen deficiency has been suggested as a cause because many affected dogs are spayed females and respond to oestrogen replacement. However, other factors are likely to be involved since not all affected dogs are female, not all dogs respond to oestrogen, and many years can elapse between ovariohysterectomy and the onset of incontinence. Phenylpropanolamine (1.5 mg/kg, three times daily) is successful in resolving incontinence in most dogs with urethral incompetence. This drug, an alpha-adrenergic agonist, works by increasing smooth muscle tone in the urethra. Other alpha-adrenergic agents that can be used are ephedrine and phenylephrine. Oestrogen therapy works by increasing the sensitivity of receptors, but is less effective and has the potential for more serious side-effects compared to adrenergic therapy.

### References
Richter KP, Ling GV. Clinical response and urethral pressure profile changes after phenylpropanolamine in dogs with primary sphincter incompetence. *J Am Vet Med Assn* 1985; **187**: 605–611.
Arnold S. Relationship of incontinence to neutering. In: Kirk RW, Bonagura JD (eds). *Current Veterinary Therapy XI*. Philadelphia: Saunders, 1992: 875–877.
Krawiec DR, Rubin SI. Urinary incontinence in geriatric dogs. *Compend Contin Educat Pract Vet* 1985; **7b**: 557–563.

**54** Indications for therapeutic monitoring of serum phenobarbitone concentrations:
• Evidence of phenobarbitone toxicity, such as such as lethargy, ataxia, or signs of liver disease.
• Poor seizure control.
• Two weeks after starting therapy to assess what concentrations have been achieved and when steady state serum concentrations are expected.
• Two weeks after a change in dose.

# 55–58: Questions

**55** What sensory nerve of the thoracic limb is being tested?

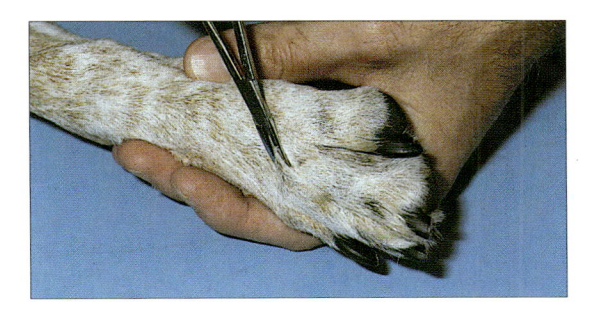

**56** What is the Schiff-Sherrington sign (**right**), and what does it indicate?

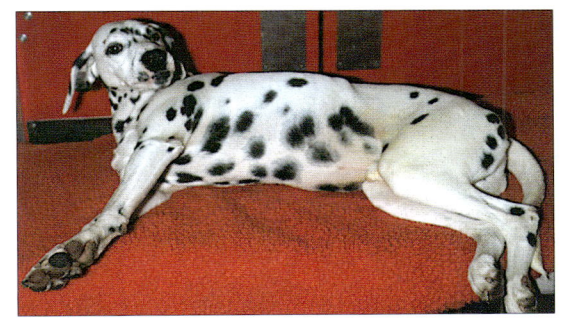

**57** These figures (**below**) illustrate the technique for biopsy of the common peroneal nerve. What are the indications for nerve biopsy?

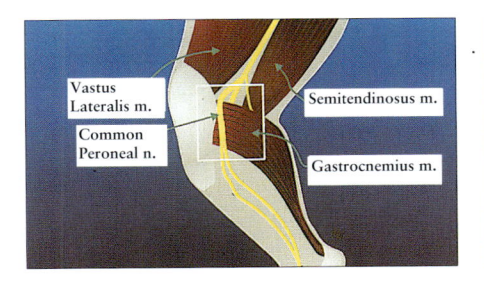

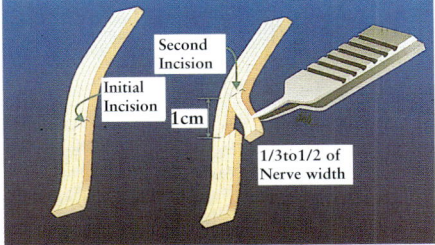

**58** This radiograph is of a four-year-old male Golden retriever with a two week duration of thoracolumbar pain and no neurological deficits.
i. What is the radiographic diagnosis?
ii. What other diagnostic procedures are indicated?

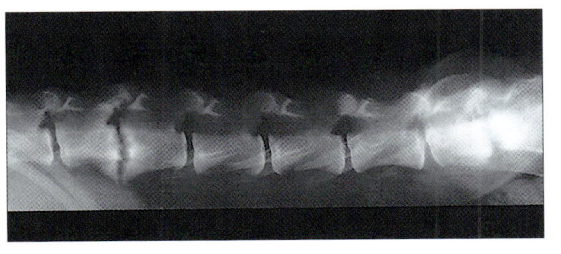

## 55–58: Answers

**55** Pinching the dorsal aspect of the paw of the thoracic limb tests sensory function of the radial nerve.

**Reference**
Bailey CS, Kitchell RL. Cutaneous sensory testing in the dog. *J Vet Internal Med* 1987; **1**: 128–135.

**56** The Schiff-Sherrington sign is seen in some paraplegic dogs, and is characterised by increased muscle tone and hyperextension of the thoracic limbs. Thoracic spinal cord lesions may interfere with inhibitory neurons, whose cell bodies are in the cranial lumbar spinal cord segments and whose axons project cranially to inhibit the thoracic limb extensor muscles.

**57** Indications for nerve biopsy are clinical signs of generalized peripheral neuropathy, such as tetraparesis with decreased conscious proprioception (CP) and weak or absent spinal cord reflexes. Electrodiagnostic studies should precede nerve biopsy.

**58 i.** Discospondylitis. There is a lysis of the vertebral endplates adjacent to the L1/L2 and L7/S1 intervertebral disc spaces. The affected disc spaces are narrowed with associated spondylosis.
**ii.** Blood and urine should be collected for culture in an attempt to isolate a causative organism. Organisms isolated from blood usually reflect the causative organism of discospondylitis. Any dog with discospondylitis should also be tested for *Brucella canis* infection in areas where the disease is endemic.

## 59–61: Questions

**59** Cultures of blood and urine from the dog in Q58 were negative. A rapid slide agglutination test and an agar gel immunodiffusion test for *Brucella canis* were positive. What do you recommend?

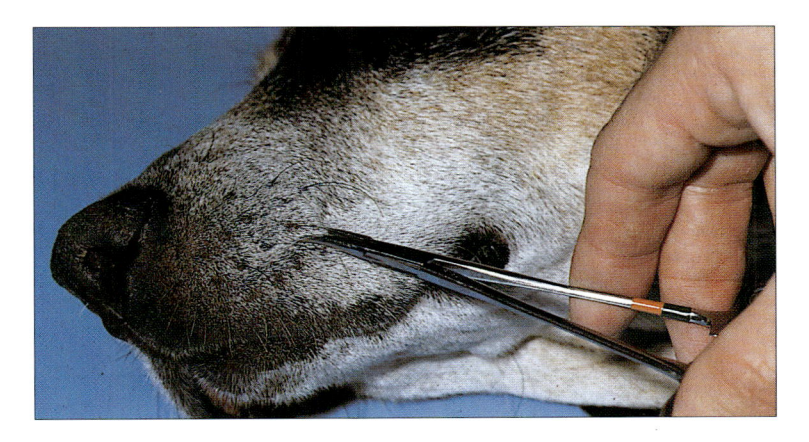

**60** What sensory nerve is being tested (**above**)?

**61** This duck (**right**) is presented for neurological evaluation. Several ducks in this flock have recently died with similar signs. Examination reveals flaccid paralysis of the pelvic limbs, wings, and cervical musculature. The bird appears alert and has normal pain perception. What is the tentative diagnosis?

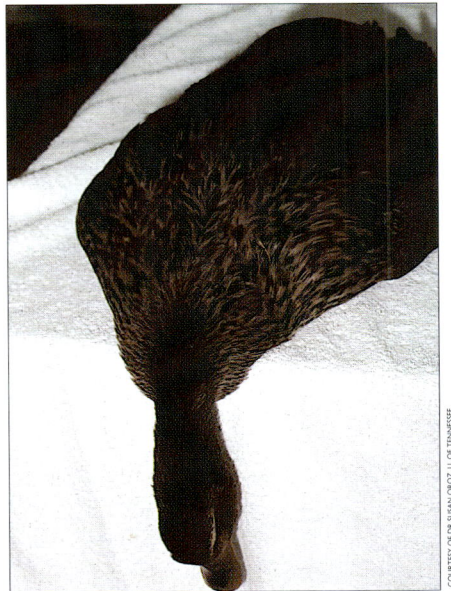

# 59–61: Answers

**59** *Brucella canis* is implicated as the causative organism in approximately 8–10% of dogs with discospondylitis in the USA. The rapid slide agglutination test is a good screening test, but the agar gel immunodiffusion test is more specific. Tetracycline in combination with streptomycin is recommended for the treatment of canine brucellosis. Fluoroquinolones may be an effective alternative (Kerwin et al, 1992). Medical treatment is usually effective in resolving clinical signs, but may not clear the dog of infection. Castration should also be recommended. The zoonotic potential of *B. canis* appears to be low, but human infection is possible.

### References
Kornegay JN, Barber DL. Diskospondylitis in dogs. *J Am Vet Med Assn* 1980; **177**: 337–341.
Kerwin SC, Lewis DD, Hribernik TN *et al*. Diskospondylitis associated with *Brucella canis* infection in dogs: 14 cases (1980–1991). *J Am Vet Med Assn* 1992; **201**: 1253–1257.

**60** Pinching the skin of the upper lip lateral to the upper canine tooth tests the maxillary branch of the trigeminal nerve. The vestibule of the nostril is often used in sensory testing, but this area is innervated by both the ophthalmic and maxillary branches of the trigeminal nerve.

### Reference
Bailey CS, Kitchell RL. Cutaneous sensory testing in the dog. *J Vet Internal Med* 1987; **1**: 128–135.

**61** Diffuse flaccid paralysis with intact sensory perception indicates generalised LMN disease. The most likely diagnosis is botulism. *Clostridium botulinum* spores are present in the soil of many marshes. Ducks become intoxicated by ingestion of contaminated vegetation or toxin-laden larval stages of flies. The toxin interferes with the release of acetylcholine at neuromuscular junctions, resulting in flaccid paralysis. Diagnosis is by detection of the toxin in stomach contents or serum. Treatment is supportive.

### Reference
Bennett RA. Neurology. In: Ritchie BW, Harrison GH, Harrison LR (eds). *Avian Medicine: Principles and Application.* Lake Worth, USA: Wingers Publishing, 1994: 721–747.

## 62–64: Questions

**62** This dog suffered thoracolumbar spinal pain for one week. Thoracolumbar disc disease was diagnosed, based on clinical data. The dog was given dexamethasone (2 mg/kg intravenously) (for the 'spinal injury') and flunixin meglumine orally at recommended doses (for the pain). Within one day the dog was pain free and the owner allowed it to exercise. The dog subsequently became acutely paraplegic, with no deep pain sensation in the pelvic limbs. This was considered to be a worsening of the disc problem and prednisolone was administered orally. Two days later the dog developed diarrhoea and vomiting, both containing blood.
i. Comment on the treatment regime, particularly the combinations of medications.
ii. How would you take the case further, both for the neurological and GI problems?

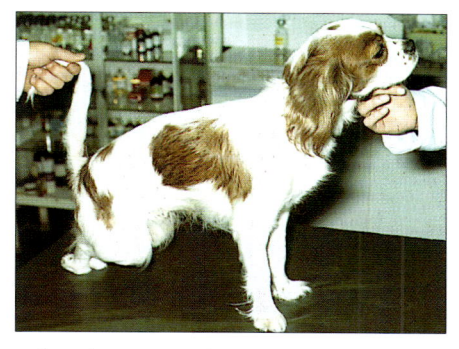

**63** In two days, the dog appears systemically ill. The rectal temperature is subnormal. The cutaneous trunci ('panniculus') reflex cut-off has moved cranially to the mid-thoracic region, and the patellar reflexes are absent.
i. What is happening?
ii. What is the prognosis?
iii. How frequently does this occur?


**64** A 12-year-old cat is presented with a six-month duration of aggression. One week prior to presentation the cat became depressed and ataxic. The cat circles to the left and postural reactions are decreased on the right. What is the neuroanatomical diagnosis?

## 62–64: Answers

**62 i.** Dexamethasone is of doubtful value in treating spinal cord injury, but its anti-inflammatory properties reduce pain in disc disease. While this may make the animal more comfortable, it may lead to increased activity, causing further herniation of disc and development of severe neurological deficits. A high proportion of dogs referred for decompressive surgery have been previously treated with corticosteroids, but with no cage confinement. Anti-inflammatory medication may be withheld during initial non-surgical treatment to encourage the patient to rest.

Flunixin meglumine is a potent non-steroidal, anti-inflammatory agent. It has significant analgesic properties, again rendering the patient susceptible to further disc herniation.

Corticosteroids (particularly dexamethasone) can cause GI bleeding in as many as 15% of neurosurgical patients, with mortality rates of up to 2%. Non-steroidal, anti-inflammatory drugs also tend to cause gastrointestinal ulceration. The combination of both classes of drugs is highly likely to lead to severe GI side-effects and should be avoided.

**ii.** Misoprostol, a synthetic prostaglandin E, is appropriate for treatment of GI bleeding. Persistent vomiting requires anti-emetic therapy. The prognosis for the spinal cord injury is poor. Dogs with disc extrusions that have absent deep pain sensation for longer that 48 hours rarely recover motor function.

**References**
Strombeck DR, Guilford WG. *Small Animal Gastroenterology*, 2nd edn. Davis, USA: Stonegate, 1990.
Wheeler SJ, Sharp NJH. *Small Animal Spinal Disorders*. London: Mosby-Wolfe, 1994: 88–89, 215–216.

**63 i.** The dog has developed progressive myelomalacia ('the ascending syndrome'). There is usually a delay in onset of several days after the onset of paralysis. Profound depression, hyperaesthesia, and systemic illness are seen. There is progressive loss of pelvic limb reflexes and the level of panniculus reflex cut-off moves cranially.
**ii.** Hopeless. Euthanasia should be performed on humane grounds.
**iii.** It is seen in 3–6% of dogs with severe neurological deficits related to thoracolumbar disc disease. (See also **Q187** and **A187**).

**References**
Davies JV, Sharp NJH. A comparison of conservative treatment and fenestration for thoracolumbar disc disease in the dog. *J Small Anim Pract* 1983; **24**: 721–729.
Griffiths IR. The extensive myelopathy of intervertebral disc protrusion in dogs ('the ascending syndrome'). *J Small Anim Pract* 1972; **13**: 425–437.

**64** Left forebrain. The behaviour change and depression are consistent with a lesion of the cerebrum. Right hemiparesis and circling to the left can be caused by a lesion on the left side of the cerebrum or diencephalon.

# 65–67: Questions

**65** A CT scan of the cat in Q64 is illustrated. This transverse scan was obtained after the intravenous administration of an iodine-based contrast agent.
i. Describe the abnormalities?
ii. What is the most likely diagnosis?
iii. What treatment do you recommend?

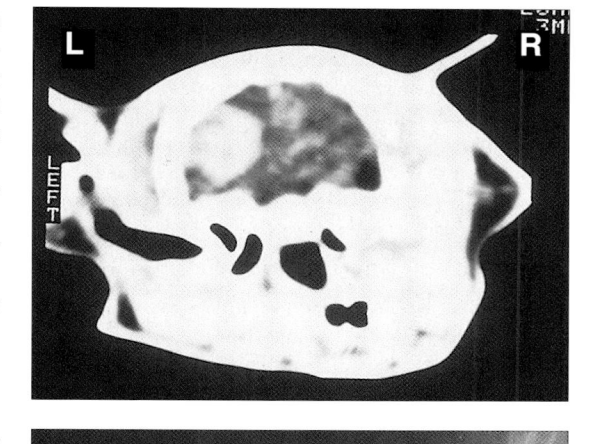

**66** The radiograph (**right**) is from a 7-year-old Dobermann with cervical pain, pelvic limb ataxia, and a stilted thoracic limb gait. The infra- and supraspinatus muscles are atrophied.
i. What is the likely diagnosis? Give reasonable differential diagnoses.
ii. Describe the radiographic findings. How dependable are survey radiographic findings in locating the lesion?
iii. What other diagnostic tests are indicated?

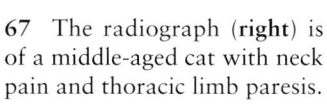

**67** The radiograph (**right**) is of a middle-aged cat with neck pain and thoracic limb paresis.
i. What is the diagnosis?
ii. What is the pathophysiology of the condition?
iii. How can it be treated and what is the prognosis?

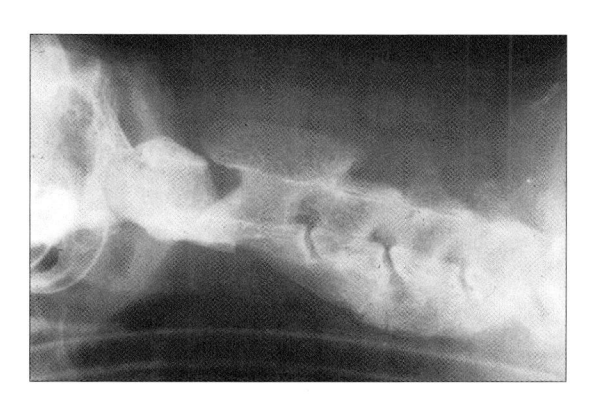

# 65–67: Answers

**65** i. There is a well-defined, hyperattenuating mass located in the left cerebral hemisphere. The mass has a broad area of contact with the skull.
ii. Meningioma. This diagnosis is based on the appearance of a peripherally located, well-defined, enhancing mass in the brain of an old cat. The entire CT scan should be carefully evaluated because multiple meningiomas can occur.
iii. Surgical excision should be strongly considered. In cats, meningiomas that are located on the lateral surface of the cerebrum can often be totally excised, and the recurrence rate is low.

### References
LeCouteur RA, Fike JR, Cann CE, et al. X-ray computed tomography of brain tumors in cats. *J Am Vet Med Assn* 1983; **183**: 301–305.
Gallagher JG, Berg J, Knowles KE, Williams LL, Bronson RT. Prognosis after surgical excision of cerebral meningiomas in cats: 17 cases (1986-1992). *J Am Vet Med Assn* 1993; **203**: 1437–1440.


**66** i. Caudal cervical spondylomyelopathy ('Wobbler's syndrome') is the most likely diagnosis. Differential diagnoses to be considered include cervical disc herniation, spinal neoplasia, meningomyelitis, and discospondylitis.
ii. There is marked narrowing of the C6/C7 intervertebral space. Survey radiographs are not particularly accurate in localising the lesion. It has been estimated that they are inaccurate in up to 35% of patients.
iii. CSF evaluation and myelography are helpful in making the diagnosis. If surgical treatment is planned, traction myelography is also useful.

### Reference
Seim HB, Withrow SJ. Pathophysiology and diagnosis of caudal cervical spondylomyelopathy with emphasis on the Dobermann Pinscher. *J Am Anim Hosp Assn* 1982; **18**: 241–251.


**67** i. Hypervitaminosis A.
ii. Severe exostosis of the vertebrae, particularly in the cervical spine, may be seen in cats fed on a diet with excessive vitamin A. Other parts of the spine and the limbs may also be involved. Clinical signs related to nerve root and spinal cord compression are seen – that is, neck pain and rigidity, ataxia, paresis of the thoracic limbs, and lameness.
iii. Treatment is difficult, but stopping intake of vitamin A can arrest the development of further exostoses, and anti-inflammatory drugs may provide relief of clinical signs.

### Reference
Clark L. Hypervitaminosis A: a review. *Austral Vet J* 1971; **47**: 568–571.

## 68–70: Questions

**68** This Dobermann experienced tenderness over the head three weeks prior to presentation. Currently, the owner complains of a prominent ridge of bone on the midline of the dog's dorsal skull. The dog has had difficulty eating. Physical examination revealed severe atrophy of the temporal muscles and a jaw which could not be opened beyond 1 cm.
i. What is the likely diagnosis?
ii. What is the pathophysiology?
iii. How would you treat the condition and what is the prognosis?

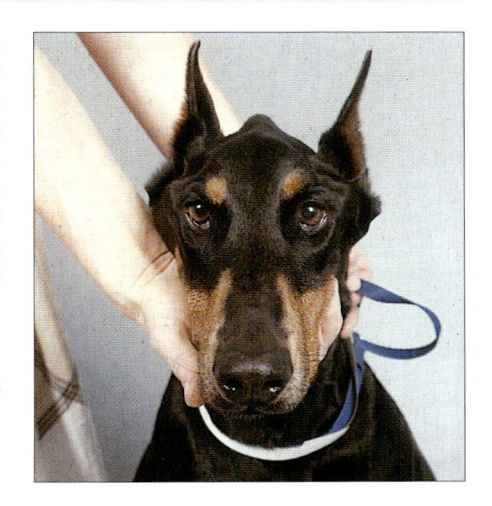

**69** This radiograph shows repair of a lumbar spinal fracture with a plate applied to the spinous processes.
i. How suitable is this as a method of spinal fracture repair?
ii. What complications may arise from its use?

**70** This photograph shows various spinal needles.
i. What are they used for?
ii. What advantages do they have over hypodermic needles?

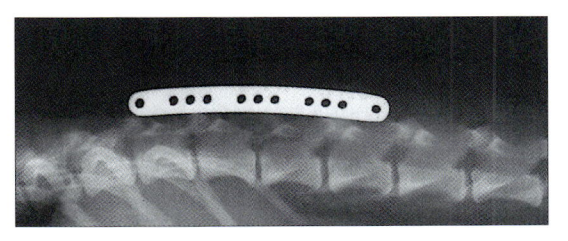

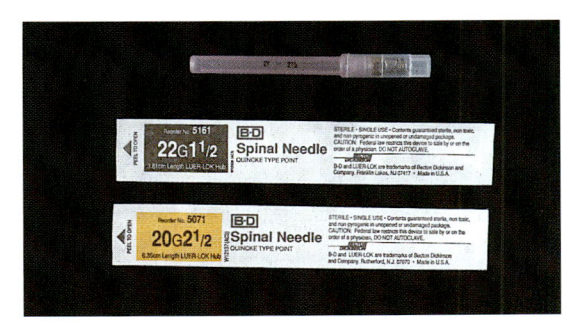

## 68–70: Answers

**68 i.** Masticatory muscle myositis.
**ii.** It is an immune-mediated disease, with circulating antibodies present directed against the Type 2M muscle fibres found in masticatory muscles.
**iii.** Treatment is with corticosteroids during the acute phase. Later, the muscles often become fibrous and affected dogs have problems opening the jaw. Many patients require continued, alternate day, low-dose corticosteroids to maintain an adequate degree of jaw movement to allow eating.

**Reference**
Shelton GD, Cardinet GH. Canine masticatory muscle disorders. In: Kirk RW (ed). *Current Veterinary Therapy X*. Philadelphia: Saunders, 1989: 816–820.

**69 i.** Not useful in anything other than small dogs and cats. Even then there are better methods.
**ii.** Dorsal methods of spinal fracture fixation have a tendency to fail, mainly because of the lack of strength of the spinous processes and their tendency to fracture and undergo pressure necrosis. These problems are greatest in the thoracic area.

**70 i.** Penetration of the subarachnoid space for CSF collection and myelography. Also, penetration of the epidural space for epidurography.
**ii.** They have a stylet, which makes blockage of the needle with a tissue plug unlikely. Also, the risk of carrying surface contaminants in the needle into the vertebral canal is reduced. The needles have a short bevel, which can more readily be positioned fully in the subarachnoid space, making epidural contrast leakage less likely in myelograms.

## 71–73: Questions

**71** This is a T1-weighted MRI image of the lumbosacral spine of a dog.
i. Describe the anatomical features.
ii. What abnormalities are visible?

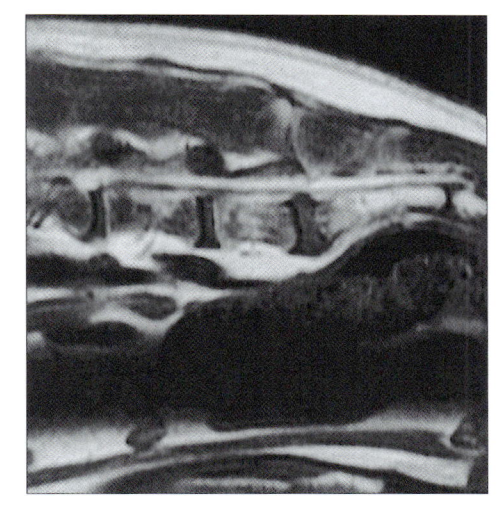

**72** What sensory nerve is being tested in this illustration?

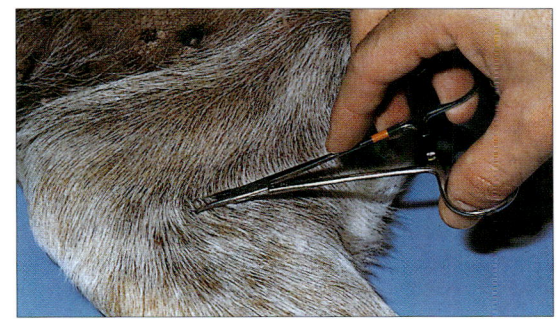

**73** A paraplegic Schnauzer is in your clinic over the weekend following intervertebral disc surgery. On Monday, you examine the dog and find this (**right**).
i. What is happening? How can it be treated?
ii. How can this situation be avoided?
iii. What early clinical signs may indicate that the situation is developing?

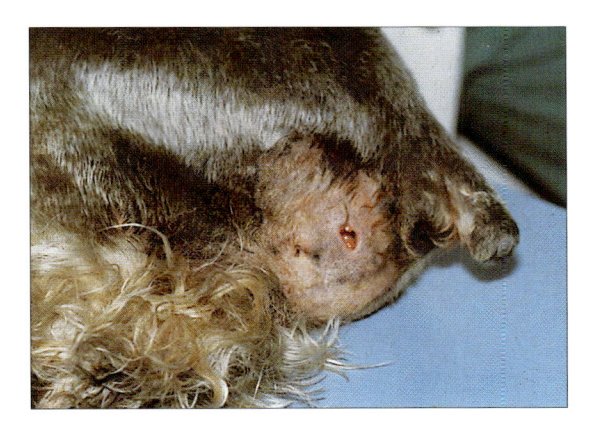

## 71–73: Answers

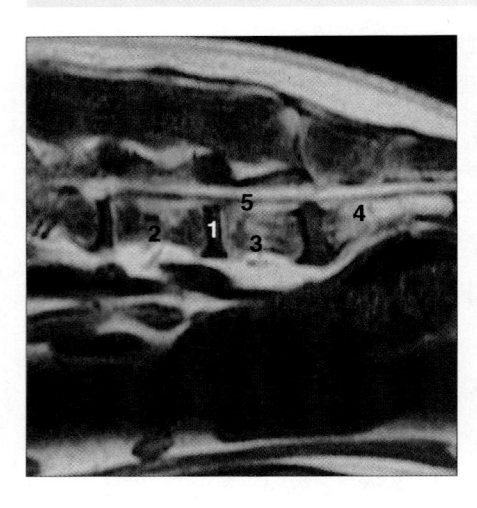

**71 i.** The following features are shown in the illustration (**left**):
1. L6/L7 intervertebral disc.
2. L6 vertebra.
3. L7 vertebra.
4. Sacrum.
5. Epidural fat in vertebral canal.

**ii.** There is dorsal herniation of the lumbosacral intervertebral disc.

**72** Pinching the skin on the medial aspect of the distal thigh tests the saphenous nerve, a branch of the femoral nerve. The saphenous nerve also usually innervates the skin on the medial surface of the paw.

### Reference
Bailey CS, Kitchell RL. Cutaneous sensory testing in the dog. *J Vet Internal Med* 1987; 1: 128–135.

**73 i.** A decubital ulcer is developing. They result mainly from unrelieved compression of tissue between a hard surface and a bony prominence. Resolution of established decubitus is difficult. Prompt removal of devitalised tissue and regular irrigation with an antiseptic solution is useful. Surgical debridement and primary closure may be required.

**ii.** The skin should be kept clean and dry at all times, and the bony prominences should be examined regularly for the onset of decubitus. An appropriate flooring material, which keeps the animal clean, dry, and free of pressure, is essential.

**iii.** Erythema, oedema, and tenderness, followed by serum exudation and alopecia. Loss of skin and subcutaneous tissue develops rapidly.

### Reference
Wheeler SJ, Sharp NJH. *Small Animal Spinal Disorders*. London: Mosby-Wolfe, 1994: 217.

# 74–76: Questions

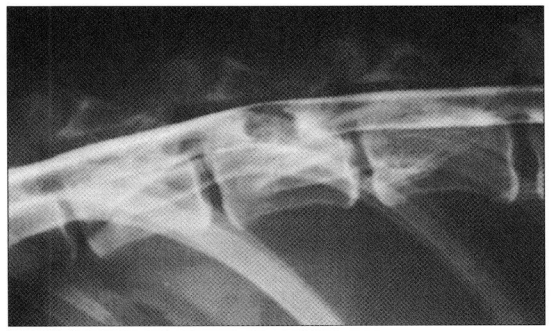

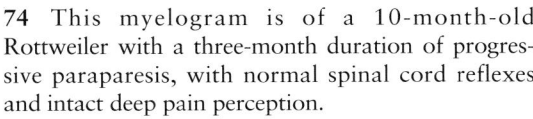

**74** This myelogram is of a 10-month-old Rottweiler with a three-month duration of progressive paraparesis, with normal spinal cord reflexes and intact deep pain perception.
i. Evaluate the myelogram?
ii. What are the differential diagnoses?
iii. What treatment do you recommend?

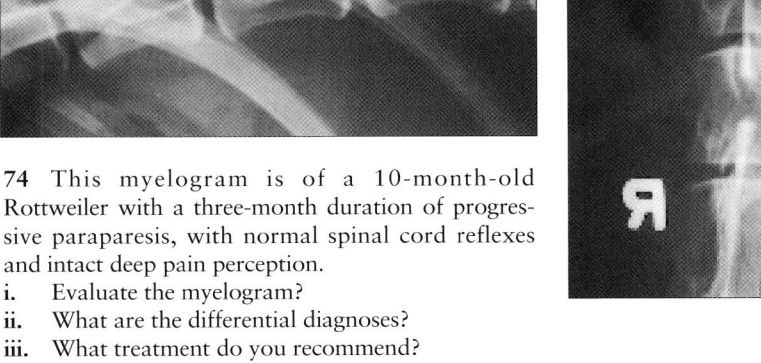

**75** What does this skull radiograph demonstrate? What are potential causes in a three-month-old Chihuahua?

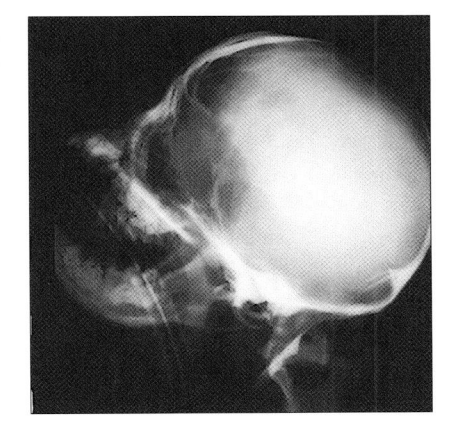

**76** A nine-year-old terrier cross has a one-month duration of depression and ataxia. The owner indicates that the dog has a one-year duration of polyuria/polydipsia and hair loss. Neurological examination shows decreased postural reactions in all limbs. Spinal reflexes and cranial nerves are normal. Laboratory abnormalities are increased alkaline phosphatase (812 iu/l), a mature neutrophilia (18,750 cells/µl), lymphopenia (615 cells/µl), and a urine specific gravity of 1.011.
i. What are the differential diagnoses?
ii. What diagnostic procedures would you recommend?

## 74–76: Answers

**74 i.** On the lateral view, there is an oval-shaped filling defect in the contrast column at T13. On the ventrodorsal projection, there is widening of the right contrast column at the cranial and caudal margins of the mass ('golf tee sign'), consistent with an intradural-extramedullary mass.

**ii.** Causes of an intradural–extramedullary mass include meningioma, nerve-sheath tumour, and neuroepithelioma. Of these tumours, neuroepithelioma is the most likely in this dog. Neuroepitheliomas typically affect large breed dogs between the ages of six months and three years. These intradural-extramedullary masses are usually located between T10 and L2. Because the cell of origin of these tumours has not been determined there is some confusion over how these tumours should be named. Authors have also referred to these tumours as epitheliomas, nephroblastomas, medulloepitheliomas, haematomas, and ependymomas (Summers *et al*, 1988).

**iii.** Surgery should be strongly considered to provide a definitive diagnosis and attempt excision. Complete surgical excision can be curative, although recurrence is common in cases of incomplete resection.

### References
Summers BA, De Lahunta A, McEntee M, Kuhajda FP. A novel intradural-extramedullary spinal cord tumour in young dogs. *Acta Neuropath (Berlin)* 1988; 75: 402–410.
Moissonnier P, Abbott DP. Canine neuroepithelioma: case report and literature review. *J Am Anim Hosp Assn* 1993; 29: 397–401.
Ferretti A, Scanziani E, Colombo S. Surgical treatment of a spinal cord tumour resembling nephroblastoma in a young dog. *Progress Vet Neurol* 1993; 4: 84–87.

**75** There is marked enlargement and doming of the calvarium. The normal features of the skull bones are lost, the structure now having a homogenous 'ground-glass' appearance. This is typical of hydrocephalus.

Hydrocephalus is classified as 'communicating' or 'non-communicating'. Non-communicating is the most common form, and is associated with congenital abnormalities in the CSF drainage pathways, meningoencephalitis, or neoplasia. Congenital hydrocephalus is seen with a high frequency in certain breeds, for example, Maltese terrier, Yorkshire terrier, Chihuahua, Lhasa Apso, Pomeranian, and English bulldog. A significant proportion of young dogs with hydrocephalus have CSF evidence of CNS inflammation and may well respond to appropriate treatment.

**76 i.** Ataxia, decreased postural reactions, and depression can be explained by a lesion in the forebrain or brainstem. The dog's hair loss, polyuria/polydipsia, and laboratory findings are suggestive of hyperadrenocorticism. If previous glucocorticoid administration is excluded, the primary diagnostic consideration is a functioning pituitary macroadenoma.

**ii.** Diagnostic evaluation should include laboratory testing of pituitary function, and CT or MRI of the brain.

## 77–79: Questions

77 Assess this contrast-enhanced CT scan (**right**) of the dog in Q76. What treatment would you recommend?

78 You are presented with a six-month-old male Yorkshire terrier. The dog is intermittently lethargic, depressed, circles, and has occasional seizures.
i. What historical information would you try to extract from the owner?
ii. What differential diagnoses do you consider likely?
iii. What diagnostic steps would you take?

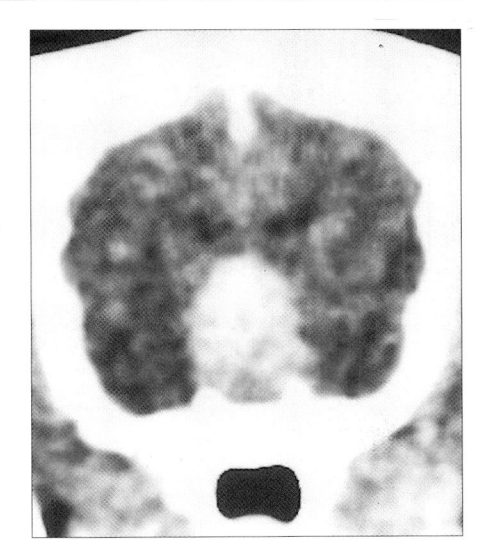

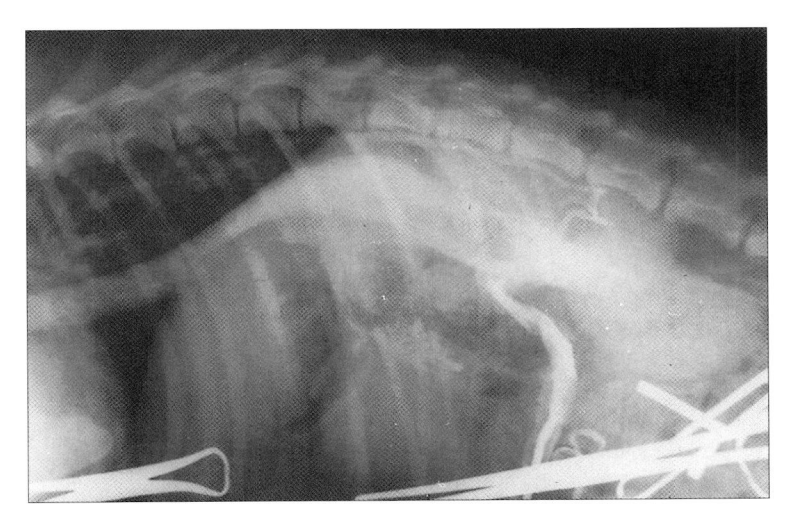

79 This is a radiograph of the dog in Q78 following surgical injection of iodine contrast medium into a mesenteric vein during laparotomy.
i. Describe the radiographic findings.
ii. Describe the various vascular abnormalities that may underlie this condition.
iii. What methods of treatment are available?

## 77–79: Answers

**77** There is a well-defined mass at the ventral aspect of the diencephalon. The lesion displays marked, uniform enhancement with contrast agent. On the basis of the location and contrast enhancement, the most likely diagnosis is a pituitary tumour. Neurological signs of pituitary adenomas and adenocarcinomas include depression, circling, seizures, behaviour changes, and blindness. Radiation therapy is quite beneficial in dogs with pituitary tumours, with a mean survival time of 740 days in one study (Dow et al, 1991). Concurrent medical therapy is often required to control signs of hyperadrenocorticism.

### References
Dow SJ, LeCouteur RA, Rosychuk W et al. Response of dogs with functional pituitary macroadenomas and macrocarcinomas to radiation. *J Small Anim Pract* 1991; 31: 287–294.
Kipperman BS, Feldman EC, Dybdal NO, Nelson RW. Pituitary tumor size, neurological signs, and relation to endocrine test results in dogs with pituitary-dependent hyperadrenocorticism: 43 cases (1980–1990). *J Am Vet Med Assn* 1992; 201: 762–767.

**78** i. Is there any previous pertinent history, particularly birth problems, vaccination status, other episodes of systemic illness, trauma, etc? Is there any pattern to the episodes, particularly related to feeding?
ii. Hydrocephalus.
Hepatic encephalopathy.
Storage disease.
Hypoglycaemia.
Encephalitis.
Toxicity.
iii. Physical and neurological examination. Retinal examination. Haematology and biochemistry, including liver function test (bile acids) and glucose, and urinalysis. Abdominal radiographs and ultrasound. Possibly CSF collection (for evidence of CNS inflammatory disease). If liver disease is suspected and portosystemic shunt is not confirmed by ultrasound, portal venography or scintigraphy may be considered.

**79** i. The portal system and hepatic vessels have not opacified. Contrast has shunted into the caudal vena cava and the azygos vein. This is an example of an extrahepatic portosystemic shunt.
ii. Shunts can be classified as follows:
• Single (congenital) – intrahepatic or extrahepatic.
• Multiple (acquired) – extrahepatic or secondary to portal hypertension.

Single extrahepatic shunts are connections between the portal vein and any systemic vein, usually the vena cava or azygos vein.
iii. Surgical attenuation or ligation of single shunts is the definitive treatment method. Multiple extrahepatic shunts may be treated surgically by banding the vena cava to improve hepatic blood flow. Medical and dietary methods of treatment (low protein diet) are also available.

## 80 & 81: Questions

80  The dog described in Q79 is treated surgically. What complications may occur after surgery?

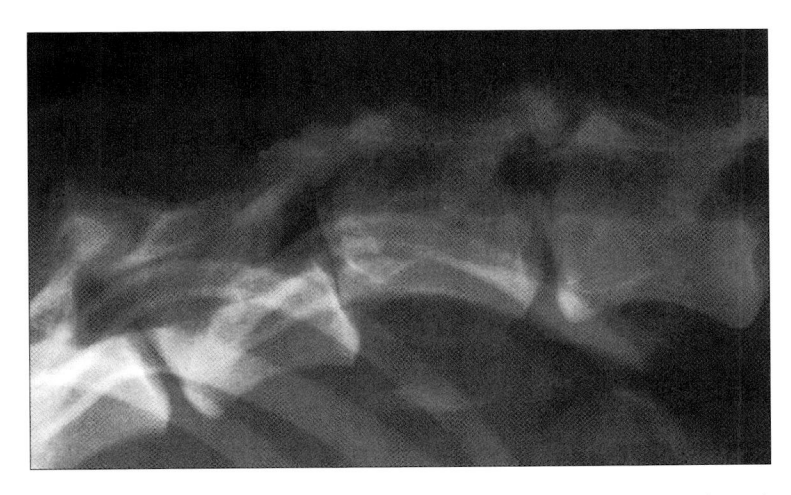

81  A dog was involved in a road traffic accident 30 minutes ago. Neurological examination reveals paraplegia with intact spinal reflexes in the pelvic limbs and intact deep pain sensation. The panniculus reflex is absent from the mid-lumbar region. There is an area of pain and swelling near the thoracolumbar junction.
i.   Localise the lesion.
ii.  Interpret the lateral radiograph of the thoracolumbar spine (**above**), taken conscious.
iii. Would you take any further radiographs at this time and, if so, how would you do this?
iv.  Is any medical treatment indicated for this dog?
v.   What other treatment considerations apply in the acute phase?

## 80 & 81: Answers

80 Complications of surgical treatment include portal hypertension, thrombosis, hypoglycaemia, and postoperative seizures.

81 i. T3–L3 spinal cord, the panniculus reflex, and pain suggesting a lesion at T13.
ii. There is a fracture/dislocation of the spine at T13/L1.
iii. The ventrodorsal projection is also needed, but it would not be wise to manipulate the dog excessively. This view could be achieved using a horizontal beam technique, but there are radiation safety implications for this. It is not wise to anaesthetise a dog soon after spinal injury, as systemic shock is likely and general anaesthesia could further compromise spinal cord blood flow with detrimental effects on the prognosis. It is better to stabilise the dog systemically prior to any major interventions. Similarly, acepromazine should not be used.
iv. Methylprednisolone sodium succinate is indicated. After acute injury, the blood supply to the spinal cord is progressively reduced. When the injured tissue is reperfused, massive amounts of highly reactive chemicals, called free radicals, are liberated. These free radicals are especially damaging to the plasma membrane of cells via a process called lipid peroxidation. Some corticosteroids can exert a powerful protective effect against reperfusion injury by acting as free-radical scavengers.

In animals, the suggested dosage regime is an initial intravenous bolus of 30 mg/kg methylprednisolone sodium succinate, followed by 15 mg/kg intravenously 2 and 6 hours later, then 2.5 mg/kg intravenously per hour for a further 24–48 hours.
v. Once the dog has been fully evaluated, analgesia should be provided, preferably by use of narcotic agents. Non-steroidal preparations are less effective and should not be given in combination with corticosteroids.

The fracture should be stabilised with an external splint. Surgical intervention, whether decompression or stabilisation, are later considerations.

### References
Brown SA, Hall ED. Role for oxygen-derived free radicals in the pathogenesis of shock and trauma, with focus on central nervous system injuries. *J Am Vet Med Assn* 1992; **200**: 1849–1859.
Wheeler SJ, Sharp NJH. *Small Animal Spinal Disorders*. London: Mosby-Wolfe, 1994; **62**: 171–191.

## 82 & 83: Questions

**82** This dog has suffered a thoracolumbar spinal lesion – a fracture at T13/L1. It has urinary dysfunction.
i. What type of urinary dysfunction would you expect with a lesion at this site?
ii. Explain the pathophysiology.
iii. What methods of management are available? What are their advantages and disadvantages?
iv. What pharmacological manipulations may be useful?

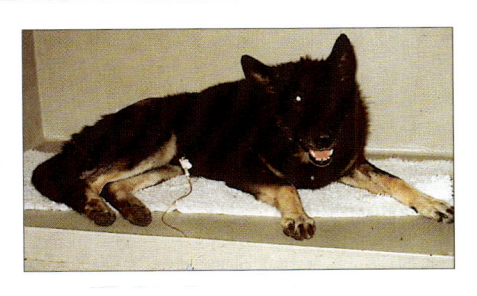

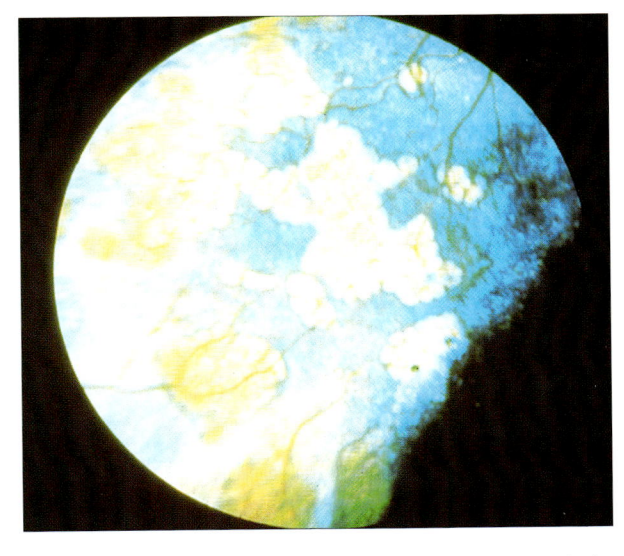

**83** A six-year-old Coonhound is presented because of a two-week duration of difficulty in walking. On neurological examination, there are decreased postural reactions on the left, a head tilt to the right, and positional vertical nystagmus. The dog's retina is shown (**above**).
i. What is the neuroanatomical diagnosis?
ii. Describe the findings on the fundic examination

# 82 & 83: Answers

**82 i.** Urinary retention and overflow – the so-called 'upper motor neuron' (UMN) bladder. The detrusor muscle is paralysed and there is increased tone in the urethral sphincter. Clinically, the dog's bladder is tense and difficult to express manually.

**ii.** The UMN bladder is seen with spinal cord lesions cranial to the sacral cord segments (**right**). The reflex controlling the detrusor muscle in the bladder wall is interrupted. Thus, afferent impulses indicating stretch in the bladder wall are not transmitted to the brain, and there is no reflex contraction of the detrusor muscle. UMNs also descend in the spinal cord to act on the urethral sphincter musculature. Interruption to these fibres causes increased tone in the urethra, as in other UMN lesions.

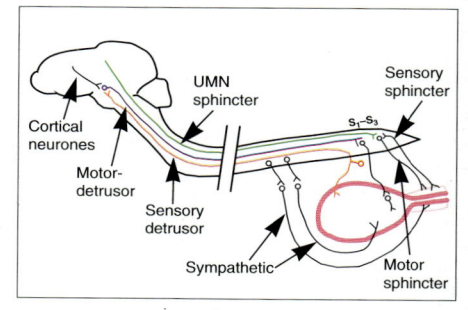

**iii.** It is important to ensure that the bladder is emptied at least three times daily, for the following reasons:
• Prevention of urinary overflow and consequent urine scald by keeping pressure within the bladder low.
• To reduce the risk of retention cystitis.
• Prevention of overstretching of detrusor muscle tight junctions.

Probably the best method for assisted voiding is simple manual expression of the bladder. However, in some patients this may not be possible. Here, intermittent aseptic catheterisation may prove necessary. Closed collection systems are useful in some patients, but are highly likely to result in urinary tract infection.

**iv.** The main problem in UMN bladder dysfunction is excessive urethral sphincter tone. It is useful to reduce the activity of both smooth and striated muscle in the sphincters:
• Diazepam (2–10 mg every 8 hours) is used to reduce the striated muscle tone.
• Phenoxybenzamine (0.5 mg/kg every 12 or 8 hours) is used to reduce the smooth muscle tone (sympathetic α antagonist). There is usually a delay of 2–3 days before phenoxybenzamine takes effect.

**Reference**
Wheeler SJ, Sharp NJH. *Small Animal Spinal Disorders*. London: Mosby-Wolfe, 1994: 210.


**83 i.** Head tilt and positional nystagmus indicate vestibular disease. Postural reaction deficits and vertical nystagmus indicate that the vestibular disease is due to a central (brainstem) lesion. With central vestibular lesions the direction of the head tilt can be to either side, but the postural deficits are ipsilateral to the lesion. Thus, the neuroanatomical localisation is the left side of the brainstem.

**ii.** There are multiple areas of hyper-reflectivity indicative of previous chorioretinitis. Such lesions are common in dogs infected with canine distemper virus, but other inflammatory diseases should also be considered.

# 84 & 85: Questions

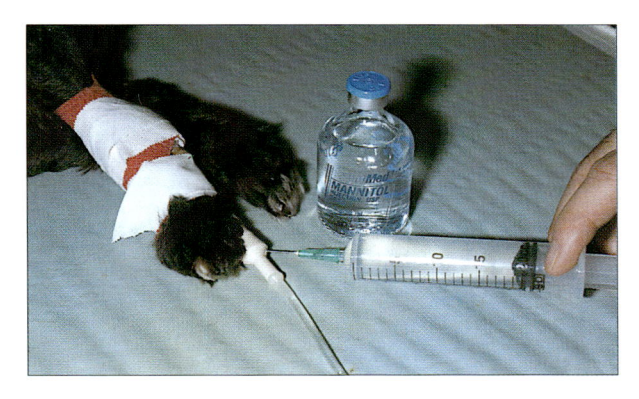

**84** What are the indications and contraindications for the administration of mannitol in neurology? What are the mechanisms of action for this drug?

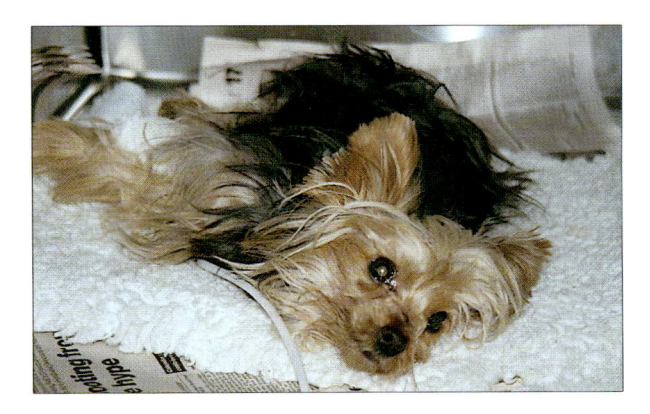

**85** This three-year-old Yorkshire terrier had been diagnosed as having idiopathic epilepsy at one year of age. Treatment with phenobarbitone had controlled the seizures, until the owner elected to cease therapy because the dog had been seizure-free for six months. It then went into a state of continual seizures – status epilepticus. The dog was presented to you.
i. What is the first priority in managing this case?
ii. How would you achieve this?
iii. What other treatment would you give?
iv. What tests would you perform?
v. What are the long-term difficulties with treating animals in status epilepticus?

## 84 & 85: Answers

**84** Mannitol is indicated in the acute management of increased intracranial pressure. Common indications include head trauma, intracranial neoplasia, and acute progressive signs associated with hydrocephalus. Mannitol is not indicated and may even be contraindicated in spinal cord injury (Hoerlein *et al*, 1983). Although many veterinary textbooks indicate that mannitol is contraindicated if intracranial hemorrhage is suspected, there are no experimental or clinical data to support this statement and mannitol is routinely used in human patients with known intracranial hemorrhage. Serum electrolytes should be closely monitored in patients receiving mannitol.

Mannitol decreases intracranial pressure by: a. increasing extracellular fluid osmolality, which reduces interstitial fluid within the brain and decreases CSF volume; b. decreasing blood viscosity, which enhances cerebral blood flow. This causes arteriolar vasoconstriction within the brain.

### References
Diringer MN. Intracerebral hemorrhage: pathophysiology and management. *Crit Care Med* 1993; **21**: 1591–1603.
Hoerlein BF, Redding RW, Hoff EJ, McGuire JA. Evaluation of dexamethasone, DMSO, mannitol, and solcoseryl in acute spinal cord trauma. *J Am Anim Hosp Ass* 1983; **19**: 216-226.

**85** i. Controlling the seizures with anticonvulsants.
ii. Place an intravenous catheter as soon as possible. Administer the following drugs intravenously:
1. Diazepam – 0.5–1 mg/kg. This can be given as a bolus. One common scenario is for diazepam to control seizures, only for them to return some time later. It is possible to repeat the diazepam. Alternatively, it can be given as an intravenous infusion, titrated to effect. (See also **Q38** and **A38**.)
2. If this is unsuccessful, give phenobarbitone – 2–4 mg/kg intravenously.
3 If this does not work, give pentobarbitone – 10–15 mg/kg intravenously. This must be given cautiously, as the previous drugs increase the animal's susceptibility to pentobarbitone. Pentobarbitone will control seizures by inducing general anaesthesia.
iii. Ensure the airway is patent and give oxygen either via a mask, endotracheal tube, or nasal catheter. Give intravenous fluids.
iv. Check the blood glucose, packed cell volume (PCV), blood urea nitrogen (BUN), and total protein. Other laboratory evaluations are less urgent, but should be acquired. Give glucose if the patient is hypoglycaemic.
v. Stabilising the animal onto maintenance anticonvulsants. If the seizures have been controlled with pentobarbitone, there is a tendency for them to occur on recovery, which may be hours or days after the initial episode. Careful administration of intravenous phenobarbitone is often required before the animal wakes up completely.

### Reference
Oliver JE, Lorenz MD. *Handbook of Veterinary Neurology*, 2nd edn. Philadelphia: Saunders, 1993: 308.

## 86 & 87: Questions

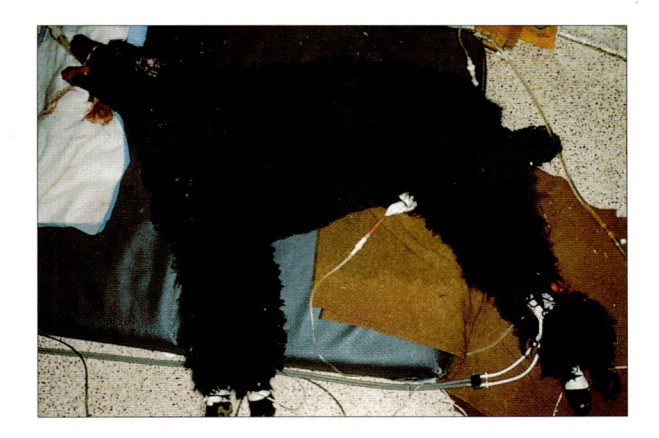

**86** This dog suffered a road traffic accident and was unconscious immediately after the incident. There is extensor rigidity in the limbs. The pupils are constricted. There is bleeding from the ear canals. Radiographs reveal fractures of the occipital condyle.
i. Localise the lesion. How does the lesion account for the dog's condition?
ii. What is the prognosis?

**87** A dog is presented with a history of head trauma. It is able to walk, but circles continually. There are lacerations over the left side of the head. You elect to radiograph the dog under general anaesthesia. One radiograph is shown.
i. Interpret the radiograph.
ii. How would you treat the lesion?
iii. You start to allow the dog to recover from anaesthesia. It has generalised seizures during this period. How would you manage the seizures?
iv. Later, the dog becomes recumbent. Locomotor function deteriorates to the extent that the dog cannot stand. It becomes stuporous. What is happening?
v. What clinical test could you perform to monitor the dog's condition?
vi. How would you manage the situation?
vii. What action that you took earlier may have contributed to the situation?

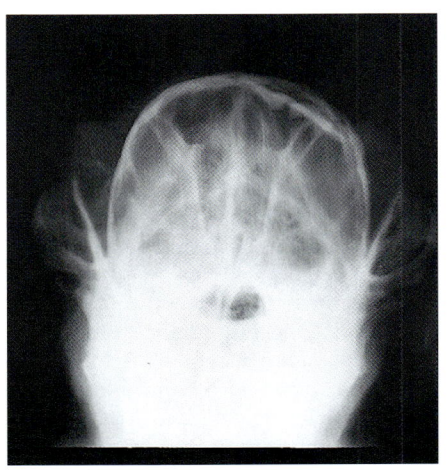

# 86 & 87: Answers

**86** i. Brainstem.
Unconsciousness – interference with the ascending reticular activating system.
Extensor rigidity – decerebrate rigidity (ie, loss of UMN inhibition from the cerebral cortex, leading to increased muscle tone in the limbs).
Constricted pupils – compression of midbrain.
ii. Poor. (See **Q30**)

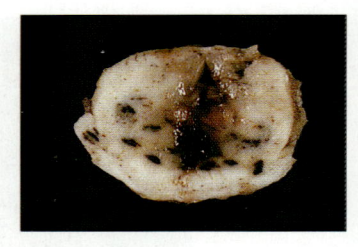

This photograph shows the brainstem of a dog that had died after a head injury, with neurological signs as described in this case.

**87** i. There is a depressed skull fracture on the left side of the calvarium.
ii. The systemic effects of shock must be managed aggressively, particularly with reference to airway, breathing, and cardiovascular function. Fluid therapy should be given. These emergency measures are particularly important in head injuries to offset the tendency of the injured brain to swell and possibly herniate. Surgical intervention should be considered in depressed skull fractures, particularly if the neurological status is deteriorating or showing signs of herniation. Use of corticosteroids in the initial phases is also recommended (methylprednisolone sodium succinate, 30 mg/kg intravenously; half dose repeated after 2 and 8 hours). Broad-spectrum antibiotics are also indicated.
iii. Administer anticonvulsants intravenously. Diazepam (0.5–1 mg/kg) as a bolus, phenobarbitone (2–4 mg/kg), or pentobarbitone (5–15 mg/kg – use with care) are all used, generally tried in this order.
iv. The intracranial lesion is progressing, probably by increasing ICP and caudal brain herniation.
v. Monitor the pupillary light reflexes (PLRs). As herniation progresses, the reflexes become progressively more sluggish, until eventually the pupils become dilated and unresponsive.
vi. Hyperventilate the dog with oxygen. This decreases the $pCO_2$, reducing cerebral blood flow and cerebral volume. Give corticosteroids as described above. If this fails to control the situation, consider mannitol (0.25 g/kg intravenously), followed by frusemide 15 minutes later. Decompressive surgery to remove depressed skull fractures should also be considered.
vii. Administering general anaesthesia. Most inhalant anaesthetics – particularly halothane – increase cerebral blood flow. Barbiturates tend to reduce cerebral blood flow, so are better choices. Also, if respiratory function is depressed, there is a tendency for increased cerebral blood flow. Some narcotics – the opioid agonists morphine and oxymorphone – also increase intracranial pressure and can depress respiration.

**Reference**
Oliver JE, Lorenz MD. *Handbook of Veterinary Neurology*, 2nd edn. Philadelphia: Saunders, 1993: 272–281.

## 88–90: Questions

**88** While vacationing in Canada, you are asked to examine a three-year-old Dobermann. The owner reports that 24 hours ago the dog seemed depressed and weak in the pelvic limbs. Now it is recumbent with flaccid tetraparesis. The dog is agitated and appears disoriented. What is the next question you ask the owner?

**89** A six-year-old male Dachshund undergoes a hemilaminectomy for acute paraplegia caused by extrusion of the T13/L1 intervertebral disc. The day after surgery the urinary bladder is distended and difficult to express manually. The dog is paraplegic with intact spinal reflexes and deep pain perception. The perineal reflex is normal.
i. What is the cause of the bladder distention?
ii. How would you treat the micturition disorder?

**90** A nine-year-old German shepherd dog has had difficulty in walking for six months. Despite aspirin administration for possible hip dysplasia the signs have progressed. The dog is ataxic in the pelvic limbs with slow proprioceptive placing (+1). The thoracic limbs and spinal cord reflexes are normal. Signs of pain are elicited on extension of the coxofemoral joints but not upon palpation of the spine. Radiographs of the pelvis are obtained.
i. What radiographic changes are present?
ii. Assess the significance of the radiographic findings.

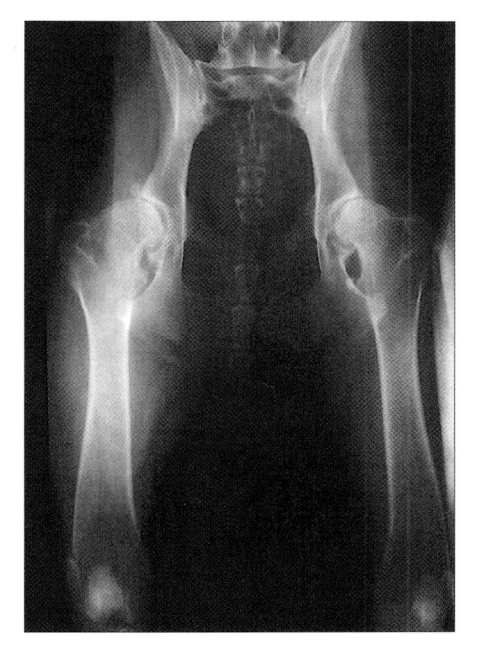

## 88–90: Answers

**88** What is the rabies vaccination history of this dog? Although the clinical signs of rabies are quite variable, rapidly progressive weakness and behavioural changes are highly suggestive of rabies. If the dog does not have a current vaccination, euthanasia and examination for rabies should be strongly recommended. Although a current vaccination does not totally exclude the possibility of rabies, vaccination failure is documented in only about 1% of rabid dogs and cats

**Reference**
Eng TR, Fishbein DB. National Study Group on Rabies. Epidemiologic factors, clinical findings, and vaccination status of rabies in cats and dogs in the United States in 1988. *J Am Vet Med Assn* 1990; **197**: 201–209.

**89 i.** The dog has UMN paralysis of the pelvic limbs and an absent micturition reflex. Normal micturition requires activation and coordination by neurons in the brain acting on LMNs in the sacral segments of the spinal cord. The difficulty in expressing the bladder manually indicates increased urinary sphincter tone, which is typical of a spinal cord lesion rostral to S1.
**ii.** Management consists of intermittent urethral catheterisation. Medication to decrease urethral tone may allow manual expression of the bladder, which avoids the risk of urinary tract infection associated with catheterisation. Phenoxybenzamine, an alpha-adrenergic blocking agent, is often effective in decreasing urethral smooth muscle tone. The dose is 0.2 mg/kg, 2–3 times daily. Diazepam (0.2 mg/kg, three times daily) is used for relaxation of the striated muscle sphincter. Bladder management should be continued until the dog regains voluntary urination. Appropriate antibiotics should be used if a urinary tract infection develops.

**Reference**
Oliver JE, Lorenz MD. *Handbook of Veterinary Neurology*, 2nd edn. Philadelphia: Saunders, 1993: 73–88.

**90 i.** There is bilateral flattening of the femoral head, thickening of the femoral neck, and subluxation of the coxofemoral joint, indicative of hip dysplasia.
**ii.** Ataxia and decreased proprioceptive placing in the pelvic limbs with normal spinal cord reflexes indicate a lesion of the T3–L3 spinal cord segments. Orthopaedic disease, such as hip dysplasia, cannot explain the neurological deficits. Animals with orthopaedic disease may be reluctant or unable to walk because of pain, but should not have decreased proprioception. When evaluating proprioceptive placing it is important to support the animal adequately. If properly performed, this test does not require the animal to bear weight on the affected limbs.

Differential diagnoses for the spinal cord lesion include degenerative myelopathy, neoplasia, chronic intervertebral disc protrusion, and myelitis.

## 91 & 92: Questions

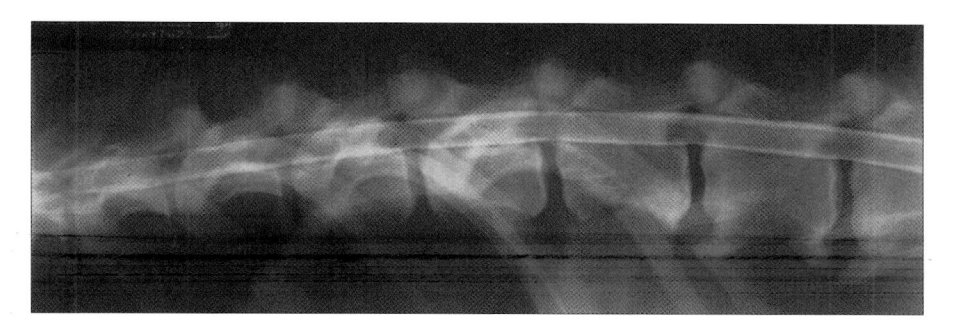

91 The myelogram (above) is of the dog in Q90. CSF examination is normal.
i. What is the most likely diagnosis?
ii. What is the treatment and prognosis?

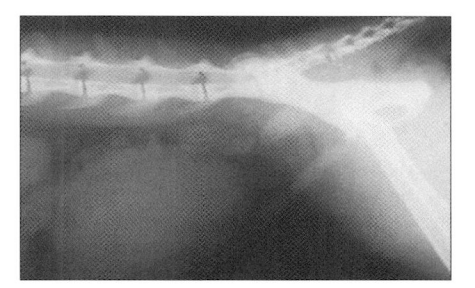

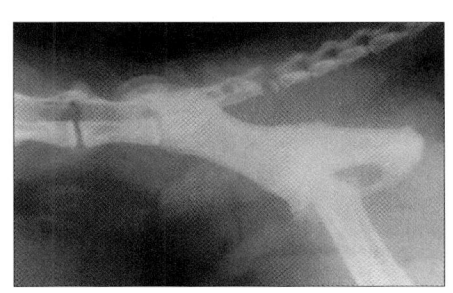

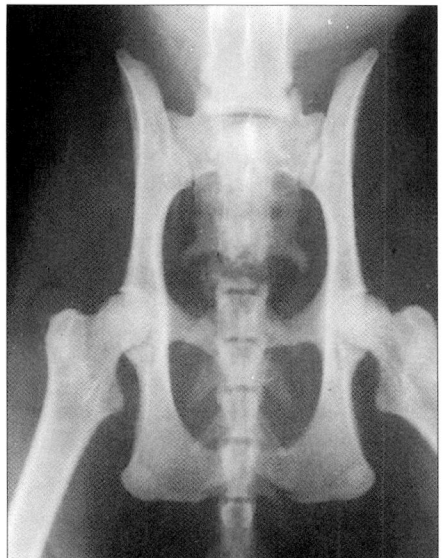

92 This cat has been in a road traffic accident. The neurological deficits appear to be restricted to paralysis of the tail.
i. Interpret the radiographic findings.
ii. What other neurological disruptions may you expect? Account for these findings.
iii. How would you manage these complications?
iv. What is the prognosis?

## 91 & 92: Answers

**91** i. The myelogram is normal. Compressive and inflammatory diseases are excluded on the basis of a normal myelogram and CSF analysis, respectively. The most likely diagnosis is degenerative myelopathy. This disease causes progressive demyelination and axonal loss of the spinal cord, especially in the thoracolumbar region. The cause is not known. Degenerative myelopathy is most common in German shepherd dogs and has an age of onset of 5–14 years. Clinical signs consist of progressive ataxia and paraparesis. Spinal cord reflexes are typically exaggerated, although decreased patellar reflexes are occasionally detected. Diagnosis is based on the typical presentation and diagnostic testing to exclude other potential disorders. Myelography is essential to rule out compressive lesions which may be surgically treatable.
ii. The clinical signs may wax and wane, but the long-term prognosis is poor. There is no treatment that has proven to be effective, but it has been suggested that the administration of vitamin B, vitamin E and aminocaproic acid (500 mg every 8 hours) along with exercise may slow the progression of this disease.

### Reference
Clemmons RM. Degenerative myelopathy. In: Kirk RW (ed). *Current Veterinary Therapy X*. Philadelphia: Saunders, 1989: 830–833.

**92** i. There is a fracture of the caudal sacrum. The urinary bladder is full.
ii. Many cats with such injuries have urinary dysfunction and, occasionally, paresis of the pelvic limbs. (Note the large bladder on these radiographs.) A lesion restricted to the caudal sacrum alone could not account for this, as the sacral spinal cord segments lie in the caudal lumbar vertebrae. In fact, there is avulsion of the sacrocaudal nerve roots from the conus medullaris of the spinal cord, caused by the traction injury that led to the fractures.
iii. The fracture itself needs no management other than possible tail amputation. The bladder must be emptied three times daily.
iv. The prognosis for return of urinary continence is favourable for cats with good anal tone and perineal sensation. However, if continence is not regained within one month, it is unlikely to occur subsequently.

### Reference
Moise NS, Flanders JA. Micturition disorders in cats with sacrocaudal vertebral lesions. In: Kirk RW (ed). *Current Veterinary Therapy VIII*. Philadelphia: Saunders, 1983: 722.

## 93–95: Questions

**93** A six-month-old kitten has been 'wobbly' since it was acquired. Neurological examination reveals an alert, bright animal, but with severe ataxia of the head and body, and hypermetria of the limbs. Cranial nerves are normal, with the exception of an absent menace response, although the cat can see. Conscious proprioception is normal, as are the spinal reflexes. There is no pain. What is the lesion localisation, likely diagnosis, and cause?

**94** In this dog (**right**) an anthelmintic was injected into the muscles caudal to the femur. It apparently suffered pain at the time of injection and immediately went lame. Subsequently, the dog was unwilling to use the limb, dragging the foot and standing on the dorsum. It continually mutilated the hock and distal limb. There were significant abrasions on the dorsum of the foot and lesions on the hock. The patellar reflex was increased. The withdrawal reflex was poor – the hock did not flex, but there was movement at the stifle and hip. Pain sensation was absent in the lateral digit but present in the medial digit.
i. What has happened here?
ii. Account for the neurological findings.
iii. What treatment, if any, is appropriate? What is the prognosis?
iv. How can this problem be avoided?

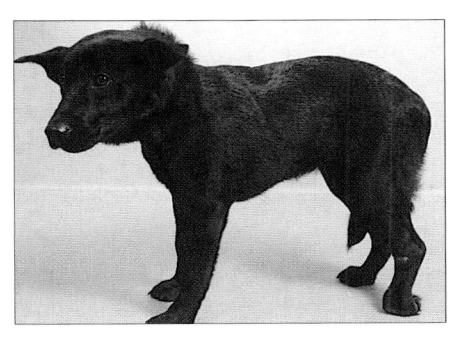

**95** A five-year-old Spaniel has suddenly been unable to close its jaw. Examination reveals a flaccid jaw, with no movement. There are no bony injuries or pain. What is the diagnosis, treatment, and prognosis?

## 93–95: Answers

**93** Cerebellum. The most likely diagnosis is cerebellar hypoplasia, related to *in utero* or perinatal infection of the dam with feline panleucopaenia virus. The virus affects rapidly dividing cells, leading to various cerebellar malformations. The pathological changes are permanent.

**94** i. The injection has been made into or near the sciatic nerve.
ii. Dragging foot and not extending digits = sciatic (peroneal) nerve lesion.
Increased patellar reflex = 'pseudo hyper-reflexia', where the muscles that antagonise the patellar reflex are damaged, giving the appearance of an increased patellar reflex.
Abnormal withdrawal reflex (poor hock flexion) = sciatic nerve lesion.
Absent pain sensation in lateral digit = sciatic sensory innervation.
Intact pain sensation medially = femoral (saphenous) nerve sensory innervation.
Mutilation of limb = paraesthesia related to peripheral nerve lesion. Animal has sensation of irritation from damaged nerve endings, and mutilates area of perceived irritation.
iii. The nerve may recover. Generally, nerves regrow at 1 cm per week, so appropriate time must be allowed. If this fails to occur, surgical debridement, removal of damaged nerve, anastomosis, or grafting may be indicated.
iv. Do not give intramuscular injections into the muscles caudal to the femur.

**95** This is probably idiopathic trigeminal neuropathy ('trigeminal neuritis'), which is a common disorder of dogs. The signs are as described in the question. There is an underlying neuritis of the trigeminal nerves, therefore corticosteroids are indicated in the early stages. Supportive treatment is also important. Atrophy of the masticatory muscles may occur and in these patients the prognosis is guarded. In most dogs recovery occurs over several weeks.

**Reference**
Braund KG. *Clinical Syndromes in Veterinary Neurology*, 2nd edn. St Louis: Mosby, 1994: 279.

## 96 & 97: Questions

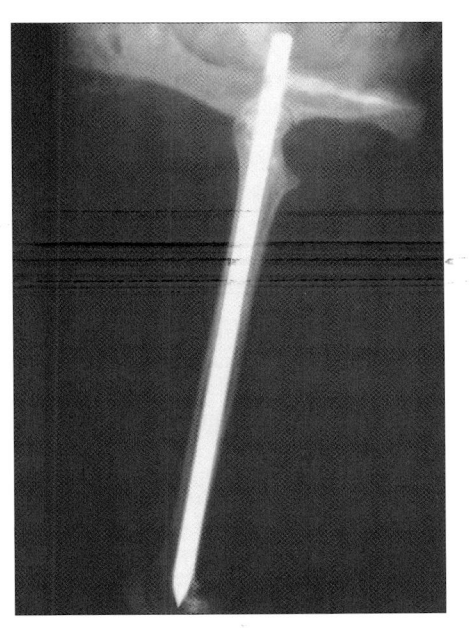

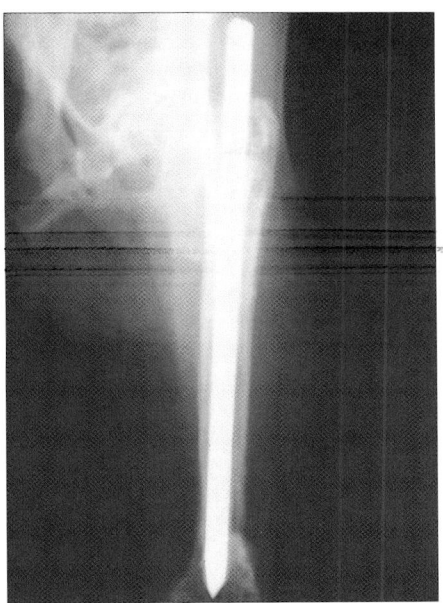

**96** You repair a fractured mid-shaft femur in a dog with two retrograde intramedullary pins. The dog progresses well until one month after surgery, when it becomes severely lame and apparently in pain. The dog is completely lame and shows a marked pain response over the greater trochanter. These radiographs are taken.
i. What is the problem and what action would you take?
ii. What is the prognosis?

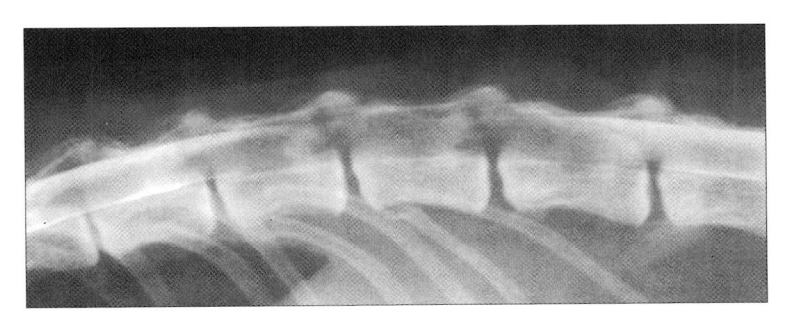

**97** The myelogram is from a three-year-old cat with a one-week duration of back pain and progressive paraparesis. Six months before becoming ill, the cat had a positive test for FeLV.
i. Interpret the myelogram.
ii. What are the differential diagnoses?

## 96 & 97: Answers

**96  i.** The pins have migrated proximally and are irritating the sciatic nerve. The pins must be removed. If the fracture has not healed, other methods of fixation must be applied. Repositioning the pins by pushing them back into place usually fails, as they migrate again rapidly.
**ii.** Fairly good with no further intervention. Sometimes, it is necessary to explore and debride the nerve. It is unusual for the nerve to be completely transected, but if this is the case, anastomosis or grafting are required.

**97  i.** There is thinning of the contrast columns from T12–L1. At the caudal aspect of the T12 vertebral body, there is ventral deviation of the dorsal contrast column, suggesting an extradural mass.
**ii.** Neoplasia, especially lymphoma, is the most likely diagnosis, although an inflammatory lesion, such as a granuloma, is also possible.
**iii.** Definitive diagnosis requires surgical biopsy, fluoroscopic-guided, fine needle aspiration of the mass, or, occasionally, finding neoplastic cells in CSF. A presumptive diagnosis of spinal lymphoma can often be made on the basis of myelographic findings, positive FeLV testing, and finding tumour cells on bone marrow cytology.

**Reference**
Spodnick GJ, Berg J, Moore FM, Cotter SM. Spinal lymphoma in cats: 21 cases (1976 - 1989). *J Am Vet Med Assn* 1992; **200**: 373–376.

## 98–100: Questions

**98** This cytological preparation of bone marrow was obtained from the cat in **Q97**.
i. What is the diagnosis?
ii. What is the treatment and prognosis?

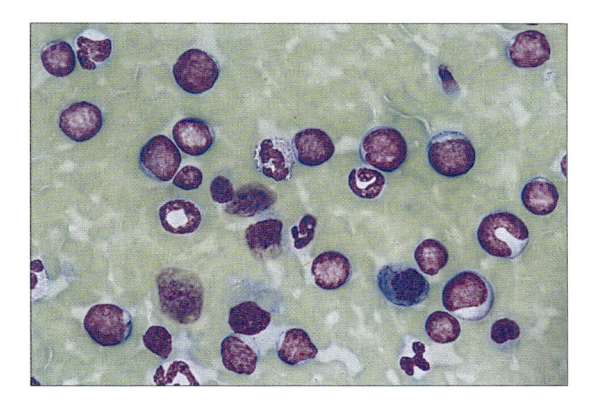

**99** This five-month-old Scottish terrier has a problem on exercise. It develops an abnormal gait mainly affecting the pelvic limbs after a period of 5–10 minutes exercise. The limbs become stiff and hypermetric. The dog is eventually unable to walk, and lies on its side with the limbs in rigid extension. After a period of several minutes, the dog relaxes. The neurological examination in the resting dog is normal. Routine laboratory findings are normal.
i. What is the likely diagnosis?
ii. Is any treatment available and what is the prognosis?

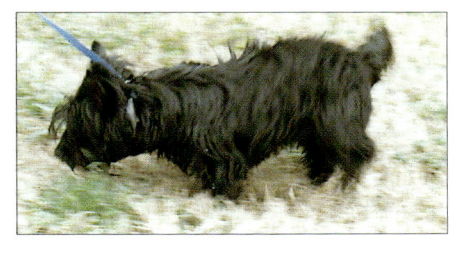

**100** What benefits does radiation therapy carry for treatment of dogs with brain tumours?

# 98-100: Answers

**98  i.** Lymphoma. Spinal lymphoma primarily affects young cats. A solitary, extradural mass extending over several vertebral bodies is the most common finding. Neurological findings usually consist of focal hyperaesthesia and rapidly progressing paraparesis. Most affected cats have detectable circulating FeLV antigen.
**ii.** Although treatment may be beneficial in temporarily reducing or eliminating clinical signs, the long-term prognosis is poor. Because most cats with spinal lymphoma have multicentric disease, chemotherapy should be considered. In one study of cats with spinal lymphoma treated with vincristine, cyclophosphamide, and prednisone, the complete remission rate was 50% and the median duration of complete remission was 14 weeks (Spodnick *et al*, 1992). Surgical excision and irradiation are other potentially useful modalities.

### References
Lane SB, Kornegay JN, Duncan JR, Oliver JE. Feline spinal lymphosarcoma: a retrospective evaluation of 23 cats. *J Vet Intern Med* 1994; 8: 99–104.
Spodnick GJ, Berg J, Moore FM, Cotter SM. Spinal lymphoma in cats: 21 cases (1976 - 1989). *J Am Vet Med Assn* 1992; 200: 373–376.

**99  i.** Scotty cramp.
**ii.** Acepromazine or diazepam may reduce the severity of the condition. The long-term prognosis is guarded.

### Reference
Braund KG. *Clinical Syndromes in Veterinary Neurology*, 2nd edn. St. Louis: Mosby, 1994: 182–183.

**100** Radiation treatment is one of several methods of treating canine brain tumours. Few brain tumours in dogs are wholly resectable surgically, therefore some sort of adjunctive therapy is desirable. Chemotherapy is one option, as is radiation treatment. In one study, radiation treatment was the most significant factor in improving patient survival time. In certain tumours, radiation treatment may be very successful – for example, pituitary adenomas. More experience is needed with the treatment of canine brain tumours, but radiation should always be considered as part of the therapeutic protocol.

### References
Heidner GL, Kornegay JN, Page RL, Dodge RK, Thrall DE. Analysis of survival in a retrospective study of 86 dogs with brain tumours. *J Vet Intern Med* 1991; 5: 219–226.
Dow SJ, LeCouteur RA, Rosychuck W *et al*. Response of dogs with functional pituitary macroadenomas and macrocarcinomas to radiation. *J Small Anim Pract* 1991; 31: 287–294.

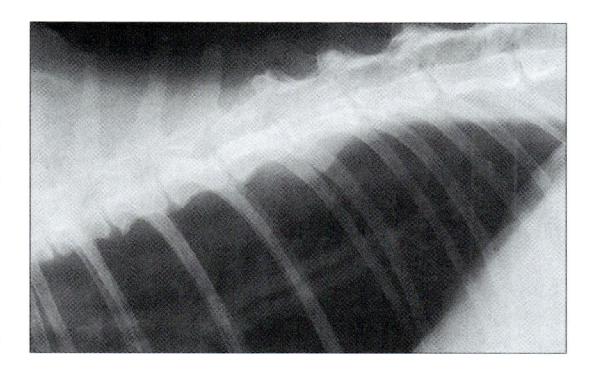

## 101 & 102: Questions

**101** You are presented with a three-year-old domestic cat. The cat has been absent from the home for one week. It was unable to walk on the pelvic limbs when the owners discovered it.
i. What conditions will you consider in differential diagnosis?
   Neurological examination reveals the cat to be severely paraparetic, with CP deficits (0) in both pelvic limbs. Spinal reflexes in the pelvic limbs are intact; the patellar reflexes are hyper-reflexic (+3). There is mild hyperaesthesia in the thoracic spine. The cutaneous trunci reflex can only be elicited in the cranial thoracic region. The femoral pulses are normal.
ii. Localise the lesion.
iii. What further tests would you perform?
iv. Interpret the lateral dorsal thoracic radiograph of the cat.

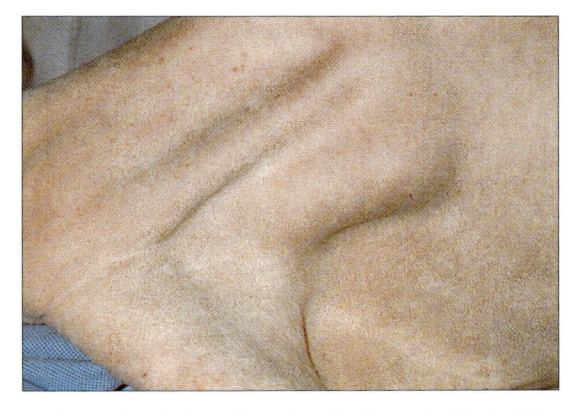

**102** This seven-year-old dog had a progressive left thoracic limb lameness over several months. Radiographic examination proved unremarkable and no cause for the lameness could be found. Latterly, the dog had become increasingly discomforted by the problem. The dog also had ptosis and miosis in the left eye, and the cutaneous trunci reflex was absent on the left side, although the contralateral reflex was intact. The dog was anaesthetised and the affected limb clipped of hair. The shoulder region is shown.
i. What is seen in the picture?
ii. What is the diagnosis?
iii. What may be found on palpation of the axilla?
iv. Account for the neurological deficits.
v. What are the treatment options and prognosis?

# 101 & 102: Answers

**101** i. Trauma.
Ischaemic neuromyopathy (aortic embolism, iliac thrombosis).
Neoplasia.
Disc herniation.
Meningomyelitis.
ii. T3–L3 spinal cord – normal thoracic limbs, UMN signs in pelvic limbs. The hyperaesthesia and cutaneous trunci reflex indicate a thoracic spinal lesion.
iii. Spinal radiographs, CSF analysis, myelography.
iv. There is a soft tissue opacity in the thorax ventral to the T10/T11 vertebrae. This may be seen in spinal lymphoma which has extended to an extraspinal location. The myelogram demonstrated this to be the site of the spinal lymphoma. Most cats with spinal lymphoma are FeLV positive on ELISA. The disease is often systemic and may be demonstrated in extraneural sites, for example, bone marrow.

**Reference**
Spodnick GJ, Berg J, Moore FM, Cotter SM. Spinal lymphoma in cats: 21 cases (1976 - 1989). *J Am Vet Med Assn* 1992: **200**: 373 –376.


**102** i. There is severe atrophy of the infra- and supraspinatus muscles, as evidenced by the prominence of the spine of the scapula. The triceps muscles also appear to be atrophied.
ii. The lesion localises to the brachial plexus and the spinal nerves that supply it. The progressive history in a dog of this age suggests a tumour. These may be tumours of the neural tissue, usually arising in the spinal nerve, termed nerve sheath tumours (pathologically classified as neurofibroma, neurofibrosarcoma, or Schwannoma). Occasionally, non-neural tumours involve the brachial plexus – for example, osteosarcoma of the proximal humerus.
iii. The tumour may be palpable either as a large mass or as a pencil-like thickening of the nerves. The latter tend to be extremely painful.
iv. The ocular abnormalities are components of Horner's syndrome – that is, interference with the sympathetic nerve supply to the eye. Sympathetic nerves leave the spinal cord in the cranial thoracic spinal nerves, some of which (T1 and T2) supply the brachial plexus.
The cutaneous trunci reflex loss is due to involvement of the nerve supplying the efferent arm of this reflex, the lateral thoracic nerve, which arises from C8 and T1 spinal nerves.
v. Poor. Amputation of the limb and tumour excision is the only option. Radiation treatment may be applied to the site. However, recurrence locally is very common. Many tumours infiltrate multiple nerves and the spinal cord early in the course of the disease. Only tumours with a long section of normal nerve proximal to the lesion, allowing full resection with adequate margins, have much chance of prolonged survival.

# 103 & 104: Questions

**103** This middle-aged, mixed-breed dog suffered a penetrating wound to the foot one week ago. A piece of wood was removed and a course of ampicillin given. Over the last two days the dog had become reluctant to exercise and stiff gaited. It had trouble eating and drooled saliva. Physical examination revealed trismus and increased muscle tone of the facial muscles and the limbs. Other neurological tests were normal.
i. What is the likely diagnosis?
ii. How would you treat the dog?
iii. What is the prognosis?

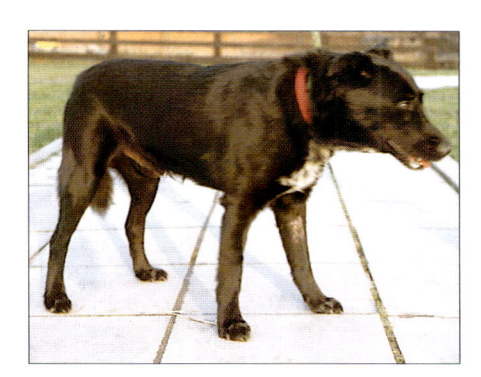

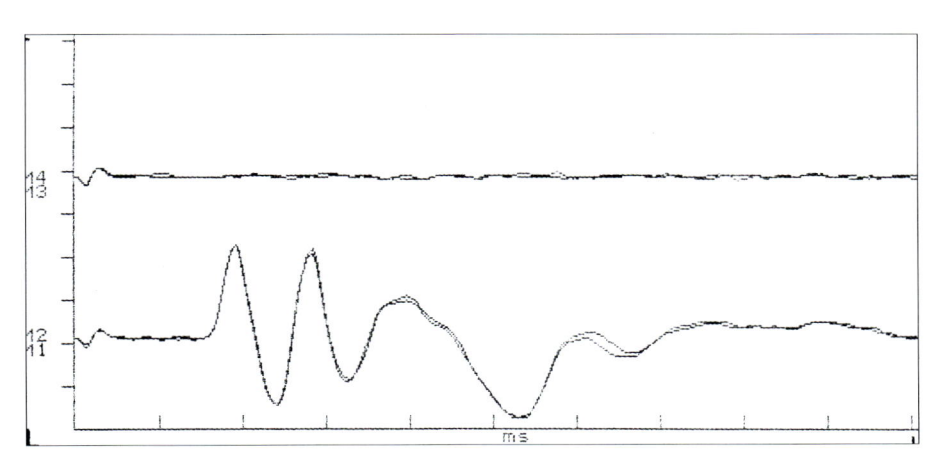

**104** A five-year-old Springer spaniel with otitis externa was anaesthetised and the ear canals cleaned and flushed with a chlorhexidine solution. Upon recovery from anaesthesia, the dog was ataxic with a head tilt to the left and spontaneous horizontal nystagmus, with the fast phase to the right. Postural reactions were normal. A brainstem auditory evoked potential test was performed. The tracing from the left ear is shown on the top and the tracing from the right ear is shown on the bottom.
i. What does the trace indicate?
ii. What is the most likely cause?

## 103 & 104: Answers

**103 i.** Tetanus.
**ii.** Give tetanus antitoxin, intravenous penicillin or ampicillin, and muscle relaxants or sedatives (methocarbamol, acepromazine, or diazepam). Try to find the site of the penetrating wound, and expose and debride it to provide aerobic conditions. Keep the dog quiet and attend to nursing requirements, including hydration and nutrition.
**iii.** Guarded.

**104 i.** Ataxia, head tilt, and spontaneous nystagmus indicate vestibular dysfunction. Vestibular disease can be due to a central (brainstem or cerebellum) or peripheral (cranial nerve VIII, inner ear) lesion. There are no other signs of brainstem or cerebellar dysfunction, so a peripheral lesion is most likely. The head tilt is toward the side of the lesion in cases of peripheral vestibular disease, so this dog's lesion is on the left.

The brainstem auditory evoked response is a recording of electrical activity in the auditory pathways elicited by an auditory stimulus. The trace at the bottom of the illustration (right ear) is normal. When stimuli were applied to the left ear (top trace) no response was recorded, confirming a lesion in the inner ear.

**ii.** Many antiseptic compounds, including chlorehexidine, can cause immediate cochlear or vestibular degeneration when instilled into the middle ear. Although the susceptibility of dogs to toxicity may vary, compounds containing chlorhexidine should be avoided or used cautiously if the veterinarian is not sure the tympanic membrane is intact. Immediate irrigation of the ear with saline to remove the toxic substance may decrease the injury. The unilateral deafness is probably permanent, but many animals appear to compensate for vestibular lesions within several weeks.

### References
Mansfield PD. Ototoxicity in dogs and cats. *Compend Contin Educat Pract Vet* 1990; **12**: 331–337.
Merchant SR, Neer TM, Tredford BL *et al*. Ototoxicity assessment of a chlorhexidine otic preparation in dogs. *Progress Vet Neurol* 1993; **4**: 72–75.

## 105 & 106: Questions

**105** This four-year-old cross-bred dog has a one-week history of cervical pain and paresis in the left thoracic limb. Physical examination reveals severe neck pain and intermittent carrying of the left thoracic limb. Otherwise the neurological examination is normal.
i. What is the differential diagnosis?
ii. How would you endeavour to confirm the diagnosis?
iii. Interpret the findings of the lateral survey radiograph and myelogram (**below**).
iv. What treatment options exist?
v. What is the prognosis, depending on each treatment method?

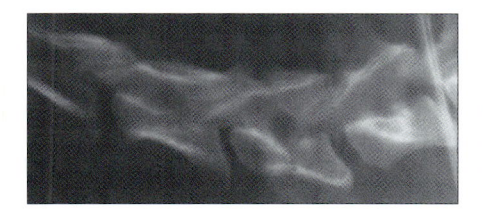

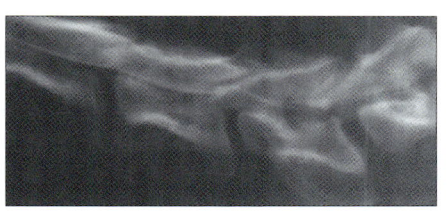

**106** This seven-year-old English Mastiff (**right**) has suffered an acute onset of weakness of the facial muscles.
i. What nerve is involved in this condition?
ii. What are the main causes of this problem?
iii. What other tests would you perform?

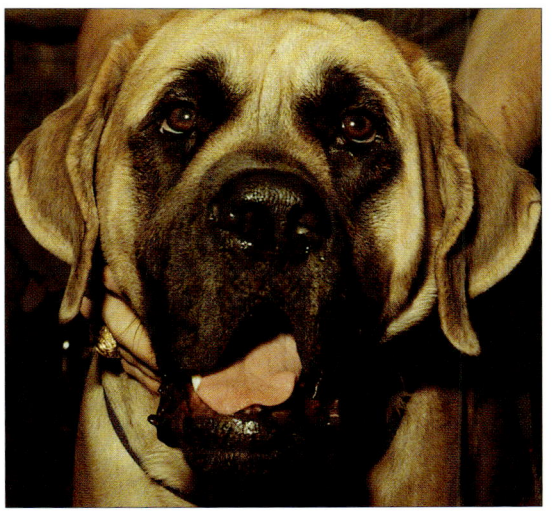

# 105 & 106: Answers

**105 i.** Disc extrusion; neoplasia; meningomyelitis; discospondylitis; trauma.
**ii.** Survey radiographs, CSF analysis, myelography.
**iii.** There is narrowing of the C5/C6 intervertebral space. The myelogram demonstrates dorsal displacement of the ventral contrast column. A radiopaque mass can be seen over the C5/C6 intervertebral space. Interpretation is of an extradural mass overlying the C5/C6 intervertebral space, probably due to a disc extrusion.
**iv.** Non-surgical treatment – cage rest, possibly accompanied by analgesics, muscle relaxants, and anti-inflammatory drugs. (Note that steroids and non-steroidal anti-inflammatory agents should not be used together, because the ulcerogenic potential of the two is increased with no therapeutic gain.)
Surgical treatment – ventral decompression, dorsal or dorsolateral decompression, or fenestration.
**v.** The prognosis for dogs with cervical disc herniations is generally good.
Non-surgically treated dogs may have a prolonged convalescent period and have an approximately 36% chance of recurrence of signs.
Following fenestration, recovery times vary. Approximately one third of dogs have a prolonged recovery after fenestration and occasional dogs deteriorate. Recurrences are few.
In a comparison of dogs with cervical disc disease that were able to walk prior to surgery, ventral decompression provided superior results to fenestration in all neurological parameters. Dogs recovered more rapidly and recovery rates were higher following ventral decompression. Thus, ventral decompression carries a more favourable prognosis both in terms of rate of recovery and time of convalescence.

### Reference
Fry TR, Johnson AL, Hungerford L, Toombs J. Surgical treatment of cervical disc herniations in ambulatory dogs. *Progress Vet Neurol* 1991; 2: 165–173.

**106 i.** Facial nerve (cranial nerve VII).
**ii.** Causes of facial paralysis are:
- Brainstem lesions (other signs of brainstem lesions seen).
- Otitis media/interna (other signs of otitis seen).
- Idiopathic – common.
- Hypothyroid-associated (possible relationship).
- Polyneuropathy (other nerves involved).
- Trauma – uncommon.

**iii.** Full neurological examination. Schirmer tear test – the facial nerve innervates the lacrimal gland. Ear evaluation, including otoscopic examination under general anaesthesia and bulla series radiographs. Thyroid function test.

## 107 & 108: Questions

**107** A three-year-old Golden retriever suffers an acute onset of right thoracic limb lameness while exercising. Over the next few hours it looses function in the right pelvic limb, left thoracic limb, and left pelvic limb, in that order. The owners report that the dog appeared uncomfortable at the onset of the problem. Physical examination is unremarkable. Neurological abnormalities are as follows:
- Tetraplegia.
- Absent postural reactions in all limbs.
- Spinal reflexes (see Table).
- No spinal hyperaesthesia.

|  | Left | Right |
|---|---|---|
| **Thoracic limb** | Withdrawal +2<br>Triceps +3<br>Biceps +3 | Withdrawal 0<br>Triceps 0<br>Biceps 0 |
| **Pelvic limb** | Withdrawal +2<br>Patellar +3 | Withdrawal +3<br>Patellar +4 |

i. Localise the lesion
ii. Give a differential diagnosis, in order of likelihood
iii. How would you confirm the diagnosis.

A myelogram was performed on the dog the next day (**above**). This is the lateral film; the ventrodorsal film was similar. The CSF reveals a mildly elevated protein (33 mg/dl) and a WBC count of 2 per µl.
iv. Interpret the radiographs.
v. How would you treat the dog?
vi. What is the prognosis?

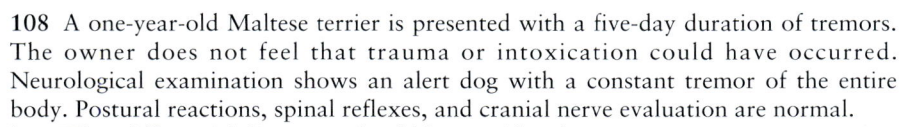

**108** A one-year-old Maltese terrier is presented with a five-day duration of tremors. The owner does not feel that trauma or intoxication could have occurred. Neurological examination shows an alert dog with a constant tremor of the entire body. Postural reactions, spinal reflexes, and cranial nerve evaluation are normal.
i. What differential diagnoses should be considered?
ii. What diagnostic tests would you recommend?

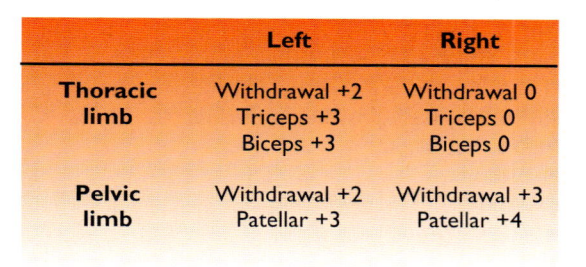

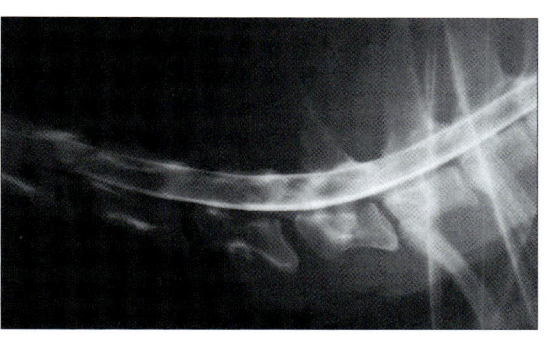

## 107 & 108: Answers

**107** i. C6–T2 spinal cord segments, mainly right-sided – LMN signs in one thoracic limb, UMN signs in the other thoracic limb and the pelvic limbs.
ii. Ischaemic myelopathy – fibrocartilaginous embolism.
Other less likely possibilities include:
- Disc extrusion.
- Neoplasia.
- Myelitis.
- Discospondylitis.
- Trauma.

iii. Survey radiographs, CSF analysis, and myelography.
iv. The myelogram is normal. This is consistent with fibrocartilaginous embolism, as are the CSF findings. Some dogs with fibrocartilaginous embolism have an intramedullary pattern of spinal cord swelling on the myelogram in the acute phase.
v. There is no definitive treatment for this condition. Careful nursing care is most important, particularly if there is urinary incontinence. Methylprednisolone sodium succinate is of benefit in acute spinal cord injury if given within eight hours of the injury, and it may be indicated here. However, prolonged use of corticosteroids is not indicated.
vi. The UMN deficits may improve, but the LMN signs are likely to be permanent.

**Reference**
Neer TM. Fibrocartilaginous emboli. *Vet Clinics N Amer, Small Anim Pract* 1992; **22**: 1017–1026.

**108** i. Acquired causes of generalised tremor include toxicities (organophosphates, hexachlorophene, bromethalin, and mycotoxins), electrolyte disturbances, and an idiopathic syndrome referred to as 'white-shaker dog' syndrome. Cerebellar disease can also cause tremor, typically an intention tremor most pronounced in the head, but other signs of cerebellar disease, such as ataxia, hypermetria, and vestibular dysfunction, are not present in this dog.

'White-shaker dog' syndrome usually affects dogs less than two years old. Maltese terriers and West Highland white terriers are most commonly affected, but a similar syndrome is seen in other breeds, including dogs that do not have a white hair coat. A generalised tremor that worsens with excitement is the most striking feature, but vestibular dysfunction, absent menace response, ataxia, paresis, and seizures are occasionally seen. A mild lymphocytic pleocytosis is usually found on evaluation of CSF.

ii. Serum electrolytes should be evaluated to rule out metabolic causes of tremor. Diagnosis of 'white-shaker' dog syndrome is based on the typical presentation and CSF findings.

**References**
Bagley RS. Tremor syndromes in dogs: diagnosis and treatment. *J Small Anim Pract* 1991; **33**: 485–490.
Bagley RS, Kornegay JN, Wheeler SJ, Plummer SB, Cauzinille L. Generalised tremors in Maltese: clinical findings in seven cases. *J Am Anim Hosp Assn* 1993; **29**: 141–145.

## 109–111: Questions

**109** Regarding the dog in Q108, results of a complete blood count, serum chemistry profile, and urinalysis are normal. Examination of CSF collected from the cerebellomedullary cistern shows nine mononuclear cells/µl (normal <5 nucleated cells/µl) and a normal protein concentration (18 mg/dl). MRI of the brain is normal. What treatment would you recommend?

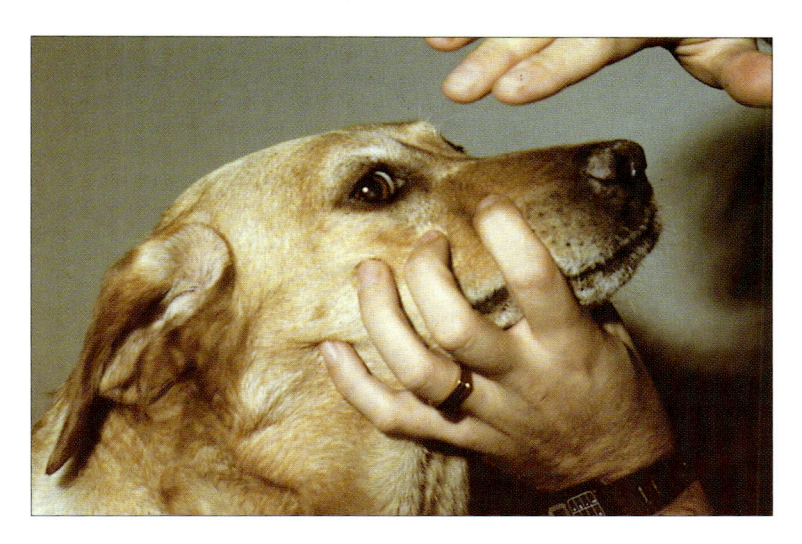

**110** This dog is having its menace response tested.
i. What is the neuroanatomical basis of the test?
ii. What other reflexes should be tested to assess any abnormilities in the menace response?

**111** A seven-year-old Cocker spaniel is presented with a recent onset of seizures. Neurological examination is normal. You starve the dog in your clinic for 12 hours in preparation for collecting a CSF sample. The dog collapses and experiences several seizures. A blood sample collected at the time of the seizures reveals a low blood glucose concentration on a dipstick test.
i. How would you confirm the low blood glucose concentration?
ii. You give the dog intravenous glucose and it recovers. The next day, the low blood glucose concentration is confirmed. What disease would you consider likely?
iii. How would you attempt to confirm the diagnosis?
iv. What is the treatment and prognosis?

## 109–111: Answers

**109** The clinical signs and findings on CSF evaluation are consistent with 'white-shaker dog' syndrome. Treatment consists of immunosuppressive doses of corticosteroids (prednisone at 2–4 mg/kg every 12 hours). The dose should be gradually tapered once clinical signs resolve. The prognosis is good, although signs may recur as the dose is decreased, necessitating another course of corticosteroids.

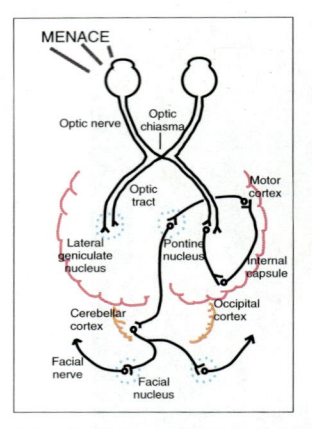

**110 i.** See illustration (left).
**ii.** Pupillary light reflex – assesses the visual pathways up to the point of the divergence of the fibres to the pretectal nucleus, at the level of the lateral geniculate nucleus.
Palpebral reflex – tests sensory function in the trigeminal nerve (cranial nerve V) and motor function in the facial nerve (cranial nerve VII), the latter also being the efferent pathway with the menace response.

**111 i.** For a quantitative evaluation, take a blood sample for laboratory analysis. If the sample is analysed immediately, a heparin tube may be used. If any time is likely to elapse, the sample must be collected into an oxalate-fluoride tube. Blood glucose declines in heparin with time, giving false results.
**ii.** Pancreatic ß-cell tumour – insulinoma. This tumour produces excess insulin in normoglycaemic animals, resulting in hypoglycaemia. Occasionally, hypoglycaemia is seen in association with other tumours, usually hepatic tumours.
**iii.** The classic test for hyopglycaemia-related neurological disease is to satisfy 'Whipple's triad' – neurological disturbance related to hypoglycaemia, fasting glucose less than 40 mg/dl, and relief of neurological signs with glucose administration. Hyperinsulinism may be confirmed by laboratory analysis of blood for insulin. Insulin concentrations are highly variable, but if the sample is taken during a period of hypoglycaemia, there should be minimal insulin in a normal animal. Abdominal ultrasound is useful, and exploratory laparotomy and biopsy are required for definitive diagnosis.
**iv.** Many of these tumours have metastasised to the liver by the time of diagnosis. However, surgical excision of isolated tumours can result in significant remissions.

In patients where surgery is not an option, medical management with prednisolone (0.25–0.5 mg/kg/day) and diazoxide (3–5 mg/kg tid) are indicated.

### References
Chrisman CL. Postoperative results and complications of insulinomas in dogs. *J Am Anim Hosp Assn* 1980; 18: 677–684.
Dunn JK, Bostock DE, Herrtage ME, Jackson KF, Walker MJ. Insulin-secreting tumours in the canine pancreas: clinical and pathological features of 11 cases. *J Small Anim Pract* 1993; 34: 325–331.

# 112 & 113: Questions

**112** A six-year-old Dobermann is presented for evaluation of a head tilt that has been present for three weeks. Otoscopic examination is normal. Neurological examination reveals a head tilt to the left and positional rotary nystagmus. No other abnormalities are detected. Laboratory evaluation detects a decreased packed cell volume (29%) with no evidence of regeneration and increased serum cholesterol (517 mg/dl). Skull radiographs are normal. What other diagnostic tests would you recommend?

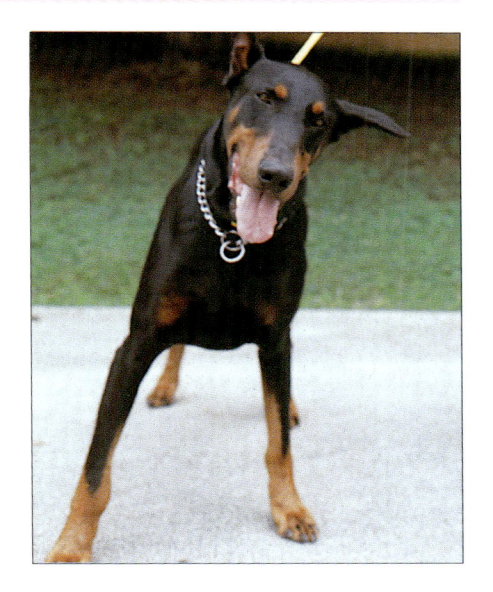

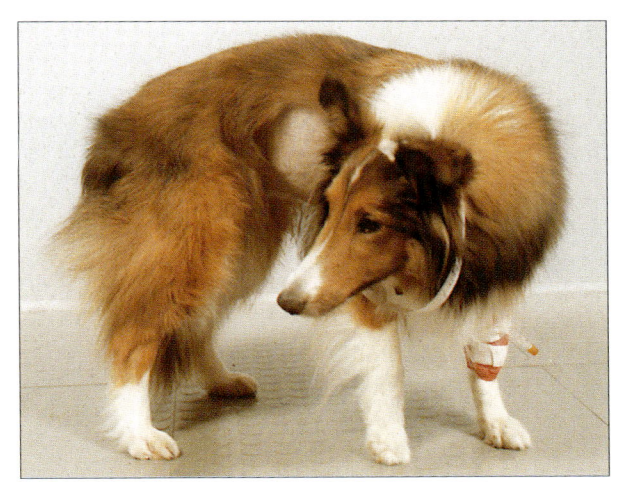

**113** This nine-year-old, previously healthy, Shetland sheepdog suffered a generalised motor seizure 24 hours before presentation. Examination reveals a depressed dog that tends to turn to the right. Postural reactions and facial sensation are decreased on the left. The menace response is absent on the left. The remainder of the cranial nerves, including pupillary light reflexes and spinal reflexes, are normal.
i. What is the neuroanatomical diagnosis?
ii. What differential diagnoses and diagnostic tests should be considered?

## 112 & 113: Answers

**112** Evaluate thyroid function. Non-regenerative anaemias and hypercholesterolaemia can occur with hypothyroidism. Various neurological problems have been recognised in hypothyroid dogs, including generalised lower motor neuron paresis, vestibular disease, facial paralysis, laryngeal paralysis, and megaoesophagus. Resolution of these signs with thyroid replacement suggests a cause and effect relationship, although the pathophysiology remains unclear.

### References
Indrieri RJ, Whalen LR, Cardinet GH, Holliday TA. Neuromuscular abnormalities associated with hypothyroidism and lymphocytic thyroiditis in three dogs. *J Am Vet Med Assn* 1987; **190**: 544–548.
Budsberg SC, Moore GE, Klappenbach K. Thyroxine-responsive unilateral forelimb lameness and generalised neuromuscular disease in four hypothyroid dogs. *J Am Vet Med Assn* 1993; **202**: 1859–1860.
Jaggy A, Oliver JE, Ferguson DC, *et al.* Neurological manifestations of hypothyroidism: a retrospective study of 29 dogs. *J Vet Intern Med* 1994; **8**: 328–336.


**113 i.** Seizures indicate forebrain dysfunction. Left hemiparesis, facial hypesthesia, hemianopia, and a turning or circling to the right indicate a lesion of the right side of the forebrain.
**ii.** A recent onset of a focal lesion affecting the forebrain suggests neoplasia or inflammatory disease. The possibility of trauma should also be assessed. Although uncommon in dogs, cerebrovascular disease should also be considered in light of the acute onset.

## 114 & 115: Questions

**114** Regarding the dog in **Q113**, results of a complete blood count, serum chemistry profile, and urinalysis are normal. MRI is performed; a transverse, T2-weighted image is shown (**right**). On T1-weighted images, the lesion is slightly hypointense with compression of the left lateral ventricle. There is no abnormal enhancement after intravenous administration of an MRI contrast agent.
i. What is your tentative diagnosis?
ii. How would you manage this case?

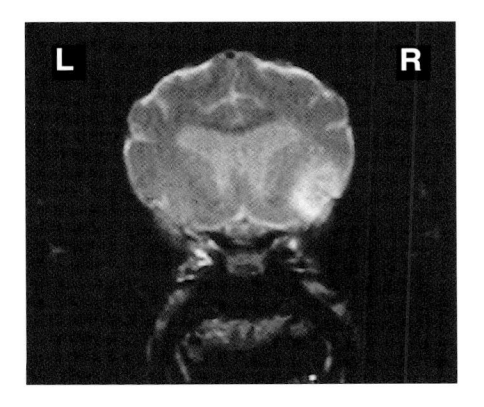

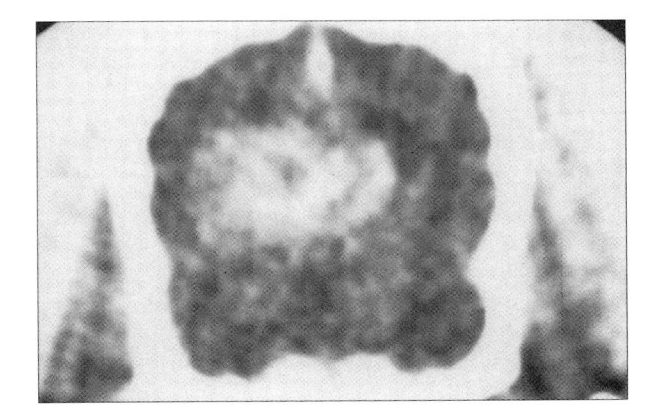

**115** This transverse, contrast-enhanced CT scan (**above**) is of a seven-year-old Boxer with generalised seizures that began three weeks previously. The dog is depressed and postural reactions are decreased on the right (+1). Spinal reflexes and cranial nerves are normal.
i. Interpret the CT scan.
ii. How would you manage this case?

## 114 & 115: Answers

**114 i.** There is a focal, hyperintense lesion involving the grey and white matter of the right cerebral hemisphere. The intensity of the lesion is consistent with oedema. The distribution of the lesion, involvement of both grey and white matter, and the lack of enhancement are consistent with acute infarction of the territory of the middle cerebral artery. Neoplasia and inflammatory disease cannot be excluded.
**ii.** Definitive diagnosis would require biopsy and histological examination. Analysis of CSF would be helpful in excluding focal encephalitis, but the mass effect evident on MRI raises the possibility of increased intracranial pressure, which may increase the morbidity associated with CSF collection. A more conservative option would be to administer glucocorticoids for cerebral oedema, monitor the neurological status and repeat the MRI in 2–4 weeks. Anticonvulsant administration is indicated to decrease the chance of further seizures.

This dog gradually improved over the course of four weeks, indicating cerebrovascular disease was likely. Cerebral infarction is considered uncommon in dogs. Clinical signs are typically acute and not progressive. Seizures, depression, asymmetrical paresis, and visual deficits commonly occur. Diagnosis is based on the typical presentation and exclusion of other potential causes on the basis of imaging (CT, MRI) and CSF analysis.

### References
Joseph RJ, Greenlee PG, Carrillo JM, Kay WJ. Canine cerebrovascular disease: clinical and pathological findings in 17 cases. *J Am Anim Hosp Assn* 1988; **24**: 569–576.
Norton F. Cerebral infarction in a dog. *Progress Vet Neurol* 1992; 3: 120–125.

**115 i.** There is a poorly marginated, heterogenous, contrast-enhancing lesion within the parenchyma of the cerebrum. The primary consideration is a glial cell tumour, such as an astrocytoma, oligodendroglioma, or ependymoma. An inflammatory lesion is also possible.
**ii.** Due to the large size, poorly-defined margins, and intraparenchymal location, complete surgical excision is unlikely. Biopsy, such as CT-guided or ultrasound-guided needle biopsy, should be considered in an attempt to obtain a histological diagnosis. Therapy with glucocorticoids to decrease cerebral oedema should be instituted immediately. Phenobarbitone administration is also indicated. Radiation therapy should be considered if the biopsy indicates glioma.

## 116–119: Questions

**116** The owners of the dog in **Q115** decline surgery and radiation therapy, but would like you to institute chemotherapy for a presumed glioma. What therapy can you offer?

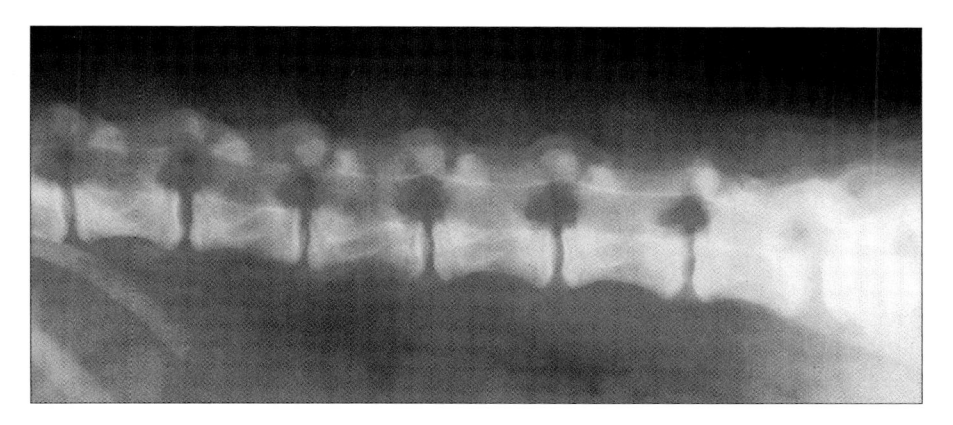

**117** An eight-month-old Brittany spaniel presents with mild weakness. You radiograph the spine and notice the irregularity of the ventral aspect of the third lumbar vertebra (**above**). What is your radiographic diagnosis?

**118** What are the three types of ataxia and what are the characteristics of each?

**119** Localise the lesion in this case: the animal is blind with absent menace responses bilaterally. The pupillary light reflexes are normal.

## 116–119: Answers

**116** The effectivenes of chemotherapy for various types of canine brain tumours has not been determined. The nitrosureas, such as carmustine and lomustine, are considered among the most effective drugs for brain tumours in human patients. Lomustine (CCNU) at 60 mg/m$^2$, orally every six weeks has been used to treat dogs with intracranial tumours (Fulton and Steinberg, 1990). The most signifigant side-effect is myelosuppression. The prognosis undoubtedly depends on the type of tumour, but in general the long-term prognosis for a dog with intracranial neoplasia is considered poor.

### References
Kornblith PL, Walker M. Chemotherapy for malignant gliomas. *J Neurosurg* 1988; 68: 1–17.
Fulton LM, Steinberg SH. Preliminary study of lomustine in the treatment of intracranial masses in dogs following localization by imaging techniques. *Seminars Vet Med Surg* 1990; 5: 241–245.

**117** Normal lumbar spine. The cura of the diaphragm arise from the body of the third and the cranial aspect of the fourth lumbar vertebrae. The ventral periosteum of these vertebrae often appears irregular on radiographs of normal dogs

**118** 1. Sensory ataxia – caused by loss of conscious proprioception from the limbs and trunk. Signs of sensory ataxia include a wide-based stance, swaying of the trunk, and knuckling and scuffing of the paws while walking. Conscious proprioception is usually tested by the proprioceptive positioning response, although an intact motor system is required in addition to the sensory system for this response. Sensory ataxia can be caused by a lesion anywhere in the afferent pathway from the peripheral nerves, through the spinal cord and brainstem, to the forebrain. Such lesions often also produce motor deficits (ie, paresis).
2. Vestibular ataxia – caused by abnormal vestibular (special proprioception) input. Vestibular ataxia is characterised by swaying of the limb, trunk, and head, with preservation of strength. Signs are usually asymmetrical, with the animal leaning or falling to one side. Extensor tone is often slightly increased. Other signs include head tilt, abnormal nystagmus, and strabismus.
3. Cerebellar ataxia – characterised by dysmetria (inability to regulate the rate, range, and force of movement) with normal strength and an intention tremor, most obvious in the head. Proprioceptive positioning is usually preserved. Other signs of cerebellar lesions may include vestibular dysfunction, extensor rigidity, absent menace response with otherwise normal vision, and mydriasis.

**119** Blindness with intact pupillary light reflexes indicates forebrain disease. The lesion must be bilateral to affect both the right and left visual pathways. Animals with cataracts may also be blind with intact pupillary light reflexes. Occasionally, the menace response is absent in animals with cerebellar disease, but other tests for vision (obstacle course, visual placing, visual following) are normal.

# 120–122: Questions

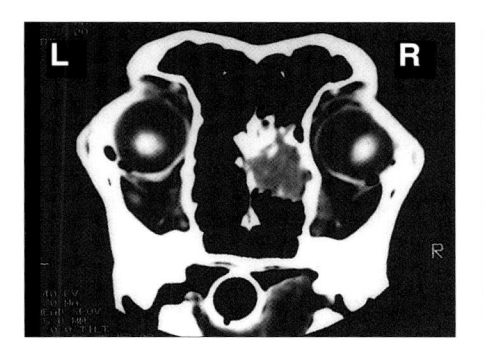

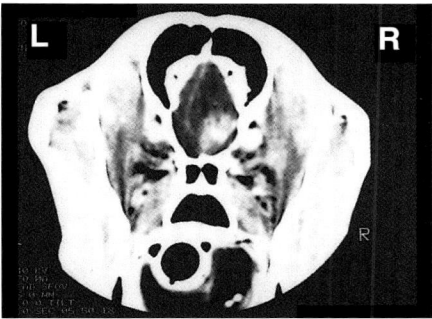

**120** A nine-year-old German shepherd dog has been treated for a persistent right-sided nasal discharge for one month. Nasal radiographs are normal. The dog develops seizures. The neurological examination is normal. **Above** are the the CT studies (following intravenous contrast medium administration).
i. Describe the CT findings.
ii. What is the diagnosis?


**121** An owner describes a seizure in which the dog becomes unresponsive, its neck flexes to the left, and twitching of the face occurs.
i. Is this a generalised or focal seizure?
ii. Why is this distinction important?


**122** You examine a six-year-old German shepherd dog with a two-week duration of progressive weakness. Neurological examination shows tetraparesis with decreased postural reactions and intact spinal reflexes. Marked signs of pain are elicited upon palpation of the cervical spine.
i. What is the neuroanatomical diagnosis?
ii. What are the differential diagnoses?

# 120–122: Answers

**120 i.** There is a soft tissue lesion in the right nasal cavity. There is a contrast-enhancing lesion in the right olfactory lobe of the brain. This is causing a significant mass effect, with displacement of the falx cerebri.
**ii.** Nasal adenocarcinoma that has invaded the brain. This is one of the more common non-neural tumours to involve the brain locally. Nasal radiographs are less sensitive than CT scanning in detecting these lesions. Lesions in the rostral forebrain may not cause neurological deficits early in the course of the disease.

### References
Foster ES, Carillo JM, Patnaik AK. Clinical signs of tumors affecting the rostral cerebrum in 43 dogs. *J Vet Internal Med* 1988; 2: 71–74.
Thrall DE, Robertson ID, McLeod DA *et al.* A comparison of radiographic and computed tomographic findings in 31 dogs with malignant nasal cavity tumours. *Vet Radiol* 1989; 30: 59–66.

**121 i.** The description is consistent with a focal (partial) seizure. Seizures may be classified as generalised or focal. During a generalised seizure there is activation of neurons on both sides of the cerebrum, whereas a focal seizure involves activation of a group of neurons within one area of the cerebrum. The most common form of generalised seizures is a tonic-clonic seizure, which is characterised by unconsciousness and extension of the limbs (the tonic phase), followed by paddling or jerking (the clonic phase). Chewing movements, mydriasis, salivation, urination, and defecation may also occur. The clinical signs of a focal seizure depend on the function of the involved area. During a focal motor seizure there is usually involuntary movement on one side of the body, as evident in this dog. Focal seizures involving the area of the brain involved in behaviour causes intermittent bizarre behaviour called psychomotor seizures.
**ii.** Classification of the seizure is helpful in determining the underlying cause. Generalised seizures can be due to a variety of causes, including primary (idiopathic) epilepsy. Focal seizures are often caused by a focal intracranial lesion, such as neoplasia, encephalitis, or vascular disease.

### Reference
Shell LG. Understanding the fundamentals of seizures. *Vet Med* 1993; 88: 622–628.

**122 i** Cervical spinal cord. Postural deficits in all limbs indicate a lesion cranial to the T3 spinal cord segment. There are no behavioural abnormalities or cranial nerve deficits to suggest forebrain or brainstem involvement. Neck pain is also localising and suggests involvement of the meninges, nerve roots, interveterbral discs, and/or vertebrae.
**ii** Neoplasia, infectious/inflammatory disorders, and disc protrusion are the primary considerations.

# 123–125: Questions

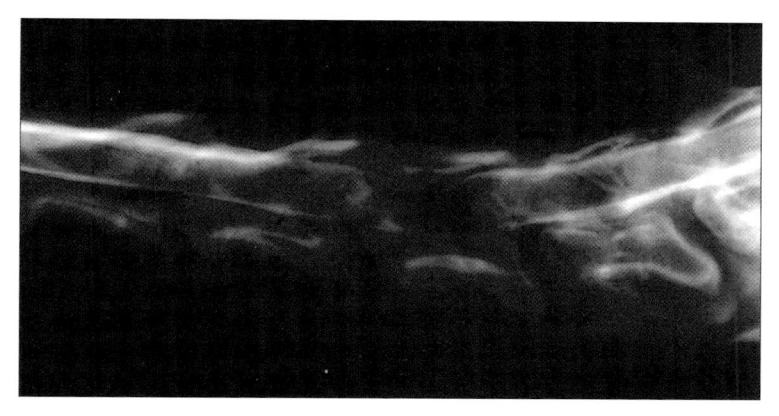

**123** The myelograms of the dog in Q122 are illustrated. What is the most likely diagnosis?

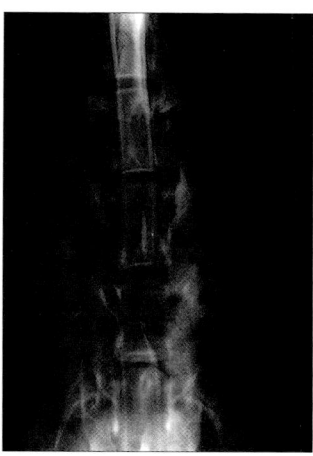

**124** Based on available scientific data, which of the following anticonvulsants are suitable for use in the long-term management of idiopathic epilepsy in dogs? Give reasons.
i. Primidone.
ii. Phenobarbitone.
iii. Phenytoin.
iv. Sodium valproate.
v. Potassium bromide.

**125** What are the indications and contraindications for CSF collection in small animals?

## 123–125: Answers

**123** There is a productive lesion, with some lysis, involving the left pedicle and lamina of the C5 vertebra. The mass is causing extradural compression of the spinal cord. A primary or metastatic tumour is most likely. The most common primary vertebral tumour of the dog is osteogenic sarcoma. Although less likely, bacterial and fungal infections should also be considered. Histological examination is required for definitive diagnosis. Vertebral tumours are rarely resectable due to the instability of the spine that results. The prognosis is therefore very poor. The histological diagnosis in this case was osteogenic sarcoma.

### References
Morgan JP, Ackerman N, Bailey CS, Pool RR. Vertebral tumours in the dog: a clinical, radiologic, and pathologic study of 61 primary and secondary lesions. *Vet Radiol* 1980; **21**: 197–212.
Heyman SJ, Diefenderfer DL, Goldschmidt MH, Newton CD. Canine axial skeletal osteosarcoma: a retrospective study of 116 cases (1986–1989). *Vet Surg* 1992; **21**: 304–310.

**124** i. Primidone is an effective anticonvulsant, but gains most of its activity from the main metabolite, which is phenobarbitone. It is more likely to have hepatotoxic side-effects than phenobarbitone, thus its use cannot be recommended.
ii. Phenobarbitone is the most effective anticonvulsant in dogs. It has a suitable half-life (approximately 64 hours).
iii, iv. Phenytoin and sodium valproate have short half-lives (two and four hours respectively), thus making them unsuitable for use in dogs.
v. Potassium bromide is generally used as an addition to phenobarbitone. It is usual to take the phenobarbitone dose to the point that the serum concentration reaches the top of the therapeutic range (10–40 µg/ml), and then to add potassium bromide if the clinical response is not satisfactory. The half-life of potassium bromide is approximately 25 days and, therefore, it is suitable as a long-term anticonvulsant in dogs.

### Reference
Schwartz-Porsche D. Management of refractory seizures. In: Kirk RW, Bonagura JD (eds). *Current Veterinary Therapy XI*. Philadelphia: Saunders, 1992:986–991.

**125** Indications:
Any patient where CNS or peripheral nerve disease is suspected, particularly:
- Intracranial lesions.
- Spinal cord diseases.
- Peripheral polyneuropathy – may be due to nerve root disease.
- Multifocal neurological diseases.
- Patients with seizures where idiopathic epilepsy is suspected, but who are not responding to adequate anticonvulsants.

Contraindications:
- Where general anaesthesia is not considered safe.
- Where there is increased intracranial pressure, as there is a risk of brain herniation.
- Where there is a fracture or dislocation at the proposed site of collection.

# 126–128: Questions

**126** How is deep pain sensation assessed? Why is it important in the assessment of animals with spinal disease? What is the neuroanatomical basis of deep pain sensation?

**127** Describe the nervous system toxicoses associated with the following drugs:
i. Metronidazole.
ii. Organophosphorous insecticides.
iii. Ivermectin.
iv. Metoclopramide.

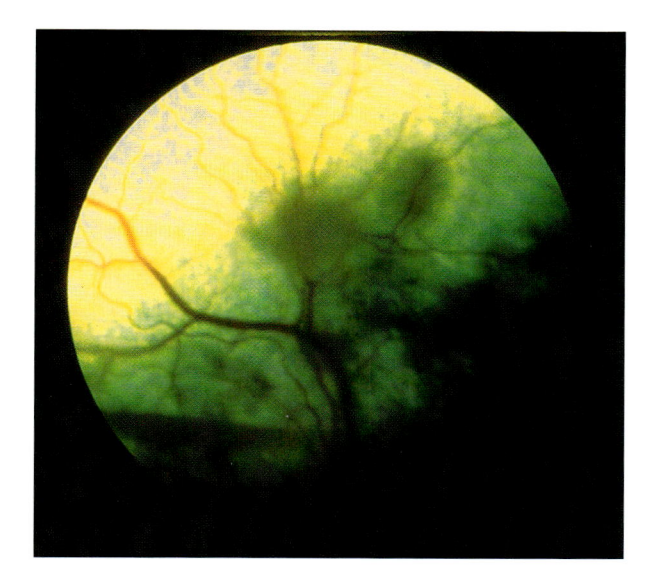

**128** A three-year-old Dachshund is presented because of decreased activity of four days duration. The owner and dog recently returned from travel in the eastern United States. Examination reveals a depressed dog with signs of cervical pain. The rectal temperature is 40°C (104°F). Several ticks are noticed on the dog. No focal neurological deficits are detected. The ocular fundus is shown (**above**). What are the differential diagnoses?

## 126–128: Answers

**126** Deep pain is assessed by applying a painful stimulus across a digit, usually with an instrument such as a large artery forceps or needle holder. If the animal has intact deep pain sensation, it will show a behavioural response to the stimulus – for example, a bark or cry. Note that simply withdrawing the foot is not an indication of deep pain sensation; it is purely a local reflex.

Absence of deep pain sensation indicates severe spinal cord damage and is a poor prognostic sign. In paraplegic dogs with disc herniations, the absence of deep pain for 48 hours or more indicates a poor prognosis even with surgery. Animals that have suffered trauma and lost deep pain sensation also have a poor prognosis.

Deep pain sensation is transmitted by non-myelinated fibres and the smallest myelinated fibres. These are the slowest conducting fibres, but are also the most resistant to compression. Also, the spinothalamic tracts and ascending reticular system, which carry pain perception, are deeply positioned and the fibres cross the spinal cord at various levels. Thus a lesion must involve most of the diameter of the spinal cord for the patient to lose deep pain sensation. This point and the fact that pain fibres are the most resistant to pressure explains why loss of pain sensation is such a severe clinical sign.

**127 i.** Metronidazole – initially anorexia and vomiting, followed by ataxia and positional nystagmus (ie, central vestibular signs). It is suggested that doses be limited to a maximum of 30 mg/kg/day, divided three times daily.
**ii.** Organophosphorous insecticides – gastrointestinal signs, salivation, muscle twitching, ventroflexion of the head and neck, generalised weakness.
**iii.** Ivermectim – gastrointestinal signs, ataxia, disorientation, seizures, depression, coma, blindness. Collies may be predisposed.
**iv.** Metoclopramide – sedation, nervousness, restlessness, movement disorders of the head and body.

### References
Dow SW, LeCouteur RA, Poss HL, Beadleston D. Central nervous system toxicosis associated with metronidazole treatment of dogs: five cases (1984–1987). *J Am Vet Med Assn* 1989; **195**: 365–368.
Neer TM. Drug-induced neurologic disorders. *Proceed 9th Am Coll Vet Intern Med Forum,* New Orleans, 1991: 261–269.

**128** The fundic examination reveals active chorioretinitis characterised by multiple areas of retinal oedema and cellular exudation. The findings of depression, fever, and chorioretinitis suggest a systemic inflammatory process. Differentials for neck pain in this dog include meningitis and discospondylitis. Disc extrusion, the most common cause of neck pain in Dachshunds, is less likely because of the likelihood of systemic disease. Tick infestation raises the possibility of a tick-borne infection, such as Rocky Mountain spotted fever or ehrlichiosis. Mycotic disease, bacterial meningitis, granulomatous meningoencephalitis, and 'steroid-responsive' meningitis are other possibilities.

### Reference
Meric SM. Canine meningitis: a changing emphasis. *J Vet Intern Med* 1988; **2**: 26–35.

## 129–131: Questions

**129** Regarding the dog in **Q128**, laboratory examination reveals hyperglycaemia (155 mmol/l) and thrombocytopaenia (50,000/µl). Radiographs of the spine show several calcified intervertebral discs but are otherwise normal. What is your next step in the management of this case?

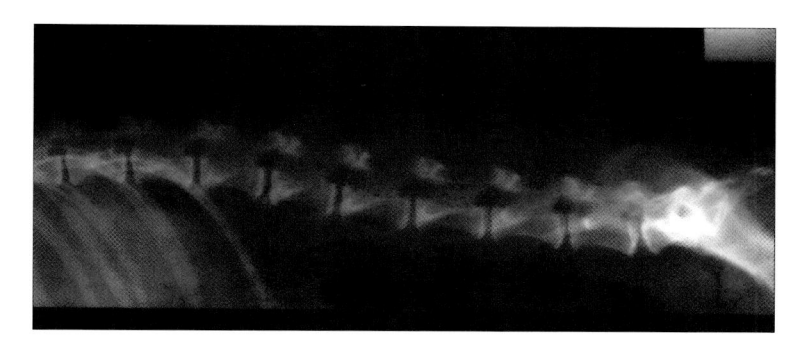

**130** Interpret this radiograph (**above**). To what disorder may this abnormality predispose?

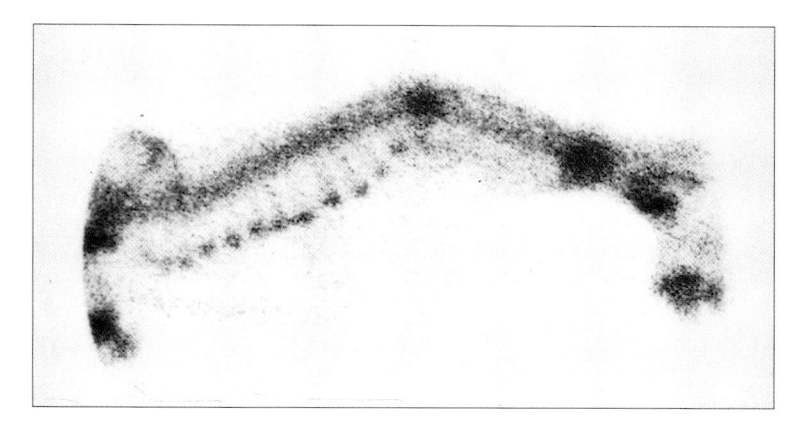

**131** This a nuclear bone scan of a dog with multifocal spinal pain (**above**). Interpret this image taken two hours after the injection of radioisotope.

## 129–131: Answers

**129** The hyperglycaemia is likely to be a response to stress. Thromboyctopaenia is common with Rocky Mountain spotted fever and infection with *Ehrlichia canis*. Both diseases can cause neurological signs, such as depression, pain, seizures, paresis, and vestibular dysfunction. Diagnosis of rickettsial disease can usually be confirmed with serology. A single elevated titre is usually diagnostic in cases of ehrlichiosis, while diagnosis of Rocky Mountain spotted fever requires documentation of a four-fold rise in antibody titre between acute and convalescent samples. Blood should be collected for serology, and treatment with doxycycline (5 mg/kg every 12 hours) or another antibiotic effective against rickettsia (tetracyclines, chloramphenicol) should be started while awaiting laboratory results. Response to therapy is usually seen within 24–48 hours but treatment should be continued for 2–4 weeks. CSF collection should be considered to evaluate for the other differential diagnoses.

### References
Comer KM. Rocky Mountain spotted fever. *Vet Clins N Amer: Small Anim Pract* 1990; **21**: 27–44.
Woody BJ, Hoskins JD. Ehrlichial diseases of dogs. *Vet Clins N Amer: Small Anim Pract* 1990; **21**: 75–98.

**130** There are eight lumbar vertebrae. The eighth is a 'transitional vertebra', having some characteristics of both lumbar and sacral vertebra. This feature can predispose to the development of lumbosacral disease.

### Reference
Morgan JP, Bahr A, Franti CE, Bailey CS. Lumbosacral transitional vertebrae as a predisposing cause of cauda equina syndrome in German shepherd dogs: 161 cases (1987–1990). *J Am Vet Med Assn* 1993; **202**: 1877–1882.

**131** There are two areas of increased localisation of the radioisotope tracer ('hot spots') in the spine: one at the thoracolumbar junction and one in the caudal lumbar area. There is a similar area in the wing of the ilium, but this is a normal finding, as this is an area of high metabolic activity. The hot spots indicate increased bone turnover, which could be associated with neoplasia or infection. Further investigations are required to make this differentiation, including radiography, blood and urine culture, and possible biopsy and culture.

### Reference
Lamb CR. The principles and practice of bone scintigraphy in small animals. *Seminars Vet Med Surg* 1991; **6(2)**: 140–153.

## 132 & 133: Questions

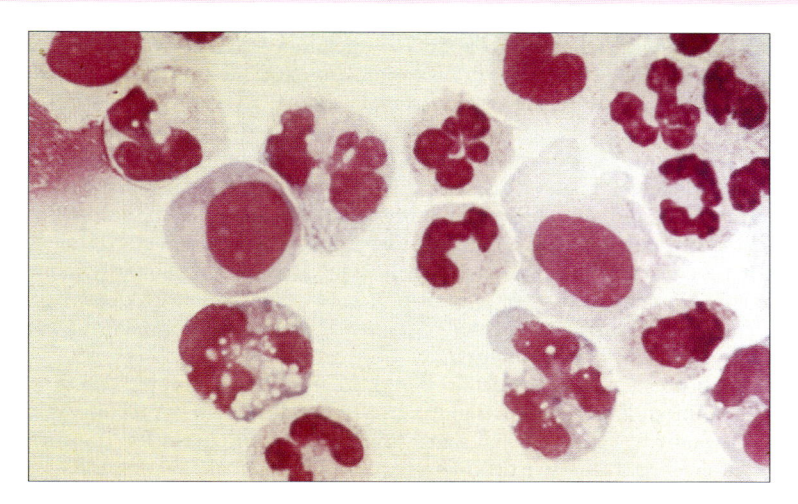

**132** A five-year-old female spayed Miniature poodle is presented with a two-week duration of neck pain. Neurological examination reveals tetraparesis with intact spinal reflexes and marked signs of pain upon palpation of the cervical spine. Evaluation of CSF collected from the cerebellomedullary cistern prior to myelography reveals increased nucleated cells (1,250 cells per µl) and increased protein (715 mg/dl). The cytological preparation is shown. What are the differential diagnoses?

**133  i.** How common is bacterial meningitis in dogs?
**ii.** Under what circumstances is it most likely to occur?
**iii.** How would you diagnose and treat the condition?

## 132 & 133: Answers

**132** Tetraparesis with intact spinal reflexes indicates a lesion rostral to the C6 spinal cord segment. The lack of signs of brain dysfunction and the presence of cervical pain further localise the lesion to the cervical spinal cord. Analysis of CSF reveals a mixed (mononuclear and neutrophilic) pleocytosis and increased protein, which are consistent with an inflammatory disorder. Granulomatous meningoencephalitis typically causes a mononuclear pleocytosis, but cases with a substantial percentage of neutrophils are not uncommon. Similar findings on CSF analysis may be seen with central nervous system infection with fungi, protozoa, or rickettsiae. Bacterial meningoencephalitis is a consideration, but usually it is associated with a primarily neutrophilic response in CSF. Canine distemper is also possible, but in mature dogs a primarily mononuclear pleocytosis is expected. Titres and cultures for infectious causes of encephalomyelitis should be submitted.

An infectious agent was not detected in this dog. Because of rapid deterioration in the dog's condition, it was euthanased. Necropsy revealed GME. A tentative diagnosis of GME is usually based on clinical signs, CSF analysis, and exclusion of other causes of encephalomyelitis. Definitive diagnosis requires histological examination.

**References**
Bailey CS, Higgins RJ. Characteristics of cerebrospinal fluid associated with canine granulomatous meningoencephalitis: a retrospective study. *J Am Vet Med Assn* 1986; **188**: 418–421.
Sarfaty D, Carrillo JM, Greenlee PG. Differential diagnosis of granulomatous meningoencephalitis, distemper, and suppurative meningoencephalitis in the dog. *J Am Vet Med Assn* 1986; **188**: 387–392.

**133  i.** Bacterial meningitis is rare in dogs.
**ii.** Infections occur most often by the following:
- Haematogenous spread.
- Following penetrating wounds.
- From adjacent septic foci (particularly the sinuses and ears).
- Iatrogenic – CSF collection or surgery.

**iii.** CSF analysis will reveal a high WBC count, mainly composed of neutrophils. Organisms may be seen on the preparation or even within WBCs, the latter being a highly significant finding. Culture of CSF is more likely to be successful if large volumes are collected and placed into blood culture bottles. If CSF provides a positive culture in the absence of a raised WBC count, this is almost certainly due to contamination.

Treatment is with antibiotics. Both the spectrum of the antibiotic and its ability to penetrate the blood–brain barrier are factors in selection. If specific sensitivity information is available, appropriate drugs should be used. Otherwise, broad-spectrum agents are used. Trimethoprim/sulphonamide, chloramphenicol, and metronidazole are suitable agents.

## 134–136: Questions

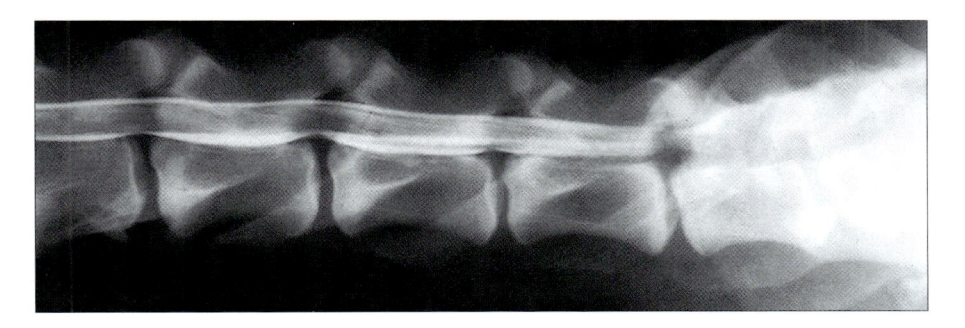

**134** This myelogram is of a five-year-old Boxer that suffered acute loss of pelvic limb function while running with the owner. Neurological examination reveals paraplegia, very brisk patellar reflexes (+3), absent flexor reflexes (0) in the pelvic limbs, and an absent perineal reflex (0). Deep pain perception is intact. Palpation and manipulation of the spine does not elicit signs of pain.
i. What is the neuroanatomical diagnosis?
ii. Evaluate the myelogram.
iii. What is the most likely diagnosis?

**135** Which of the following diseases can result in alterations of the sense of smell in dogs?
a. Distemper.
b. Parainfluenza.
c. Nasal neoplasia.
d. Diabetes mellitus.
e. All of the above.

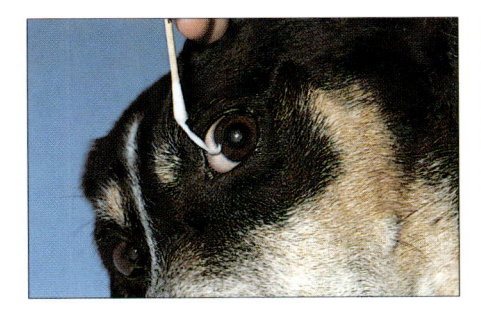

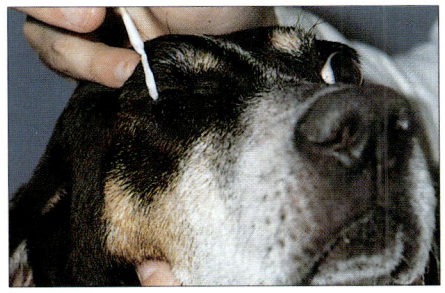

**136** Localise the neurological deficit. On touching the left cornea the globe does not retract and the eye does not blink (**above, left**). On touching the right cornea, the globe retracts and the eye blinks (**above, right**). The face is symmetrical and the dog spontaneously blinks both eyes.

## 134–136: Answers

**134 i.** There is a lesion involving the L6–S3 spinal cord segments. Absent flexor reflexes can be caused by a lesion of the L6–S1 spinal cord segments. The perineal reflex is mediated through the S1–S3 segments. Lesions involving both sciatic nerves and both pudendal nerves would cause identical signs, but would be extremely uncommon. An exaggerated patellar reflex usually indicates a lesion rostral to L4, but in this case it is due to lack of damping by the denervated flexors of the stifle ('pseudo-hyper-reflexia').
**ii.** The myelogram is normal.
**iii.** The acute onset of a focal spinal cord lesion is most suggestive of a traumatic or vascular disorder. The lack of pain on palpation of the spine and the normal myelogram exclude compressive lesions such as fractures, luxation, and intervertebral disc extrusions. Spinal cord ischaemia due to emboli of fibrocartilage arising from an intervertebral disc occurs most commonly in large breed and giant breed dogs. Clinical signs are invariably acute and may be related to exertion or minor trauma. Neurological examination reveals a focal, usually non-painful, spinal cord lesion. Asymmetrical deficits are common. Presumptive diagnosis is based on the typical history and clinical signs and exclusion of other disorders by radiography, myelography, and CSF analysis. The neurological deficits may resolve within several weeks, but permanent dysfunction is possible, especially in severe cases. There is no specific treatment other than supportive care and management of any incontinence.

### Reference
Penwick RC. Fibrocartilagenous embolism and ischemic myelopathy. *Compend Contin Educat Pract Vet* 1989; **11**:287–298.

**135 e.** All of these diseases are reported causes of alterations in the sense of smell.

### Reference
Myers LJ. Dysosmia of the dog in clinical veterinary medicine. *Prog Vet Neurol* 1990; **1**: 171–179.

**136** Ophthalmic branch of the left trigeminal nerve. The corneal reflex is initiated by lightly touching the cornea, which produces retraction of the globe and an eye blink. The sensory component of this reflex is mediated by the ophthalmic branch of the trigeminal nerve. The motor response is mediated through the facial nerve for the eye blink and the abducens nerve for retraction of the globe. This reflex is integrated in the brainstem.

## 137–139: Questions

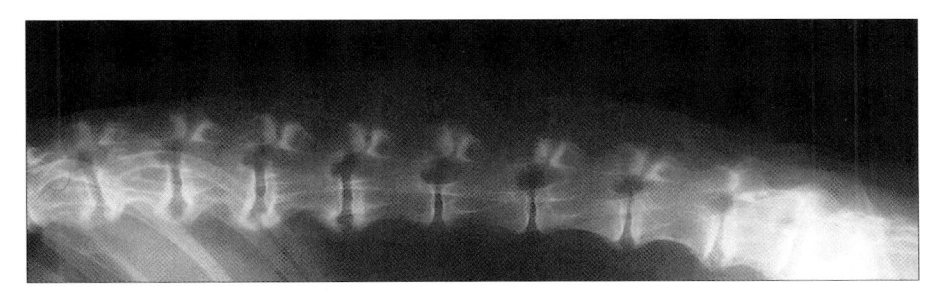

**137** This radiograph is of a 10-year-old German shepherd dog with a two-week duration of paraparesis. Neurological examination reveals pelvic limb ataxia, and decreased proprioceptive positioning in the pelvic limbs with intact spinal reflexes.
i. Describe the radiographic abnormalities?
ii. Considering the neurological findings, what is the significance of the radiographic changes?

**138** A five-year-old dog has experienced a subacute onset of flaccid paralysis over the past two days. The dog is unable to stand, although it can raise its head. Conscious proprioception is absent. There are no spinal reflexes (0) and muscle tone is poor. Deep pain sensation is intact. The owner reports that the dog's bark has altered.
i. Localise the problem.
ii. What historical information should you seek?
iii. What are the possible causes and the respective prognoses?

**139** An aged cat is presented with a progressively deteriorating ability to jump. Examination reveals poor muscle mass. The cat walks with a plantigrade posture. Conscious proprioception is poor and the spinal reflexes reduced (+1).
i. Localise the lesion.
ii. What tests would you perform to assist in the diagnosis?

## 137–139: Answers

**137 i.** There are multiple areas of spondylosis deformans characterised by sclerosis of the vertebral end plates and osteophyte production adjacent to the intervertebral disc spaces.
**ii.** Spondylosis deformans is common in older dogs, especially in large breeds. This condition is a non-inflammatory response to degeneration of the intervertebral discs. Spondylosis deformans is rarely of clinical significance. Myelography and CSF analysis are indicated to investigate other potential causes of this dog's spinal cord disease.

**Reference**
Romatowski J. Spondylosis deformans in the dog. *Compend Contin Educat Pract Vet* 1986; 8: 531–534.

**138 i.** Generalised motor unit disease.
**ii.** The dog's lifestyle and particularly whether there has been any interaction with a raccoon; if the dog has eaten any carcases; or whether any ticks have been found on it. (Obviously these questions will vary depending on the geographical region of the occurrence.)
**iii.** 1. Distal denervating disease – a degenerative process of the terminal branches of the motor nerves. Mainly reported in the UK. Carries a good prognosis.
2. Coonhound paralysis – immune-mediated reaction to raccoon saliva, causing a polyradiculoneuritis. Prognosis is good, but may require respiratory support.
3. Tick paralysis – toxin interferes with acetylcholine release at the neuromuscular junction. If the tick is found and removed, the prognosis is generally good. However, Australian tick paralysis is a severe disease, which can lead to death.
4. Botulism – intoxication by the toxin of *Clostridium botulinum* following ingestion of infested foodstuffs. This also causes a presynaptic neuromuscular junction blockade. Confirmation of the diagnosis can be difficult, but is generally by identification of toxin in serum, faeces, vomitus, or the ingested food. The prognosis is good with suitable supportive therapy.

**139 i.** Generalised polyneuropathy.
**ii.** Electrophysiology (electromyography and nerve conduction studies) to confirm the nature of the disorder. The most common cause of peripheral polyneuropathy in cats is diabetes mellitus, therefore blood and urine glucose analysis is indicated.

## 140 & 141: Questions

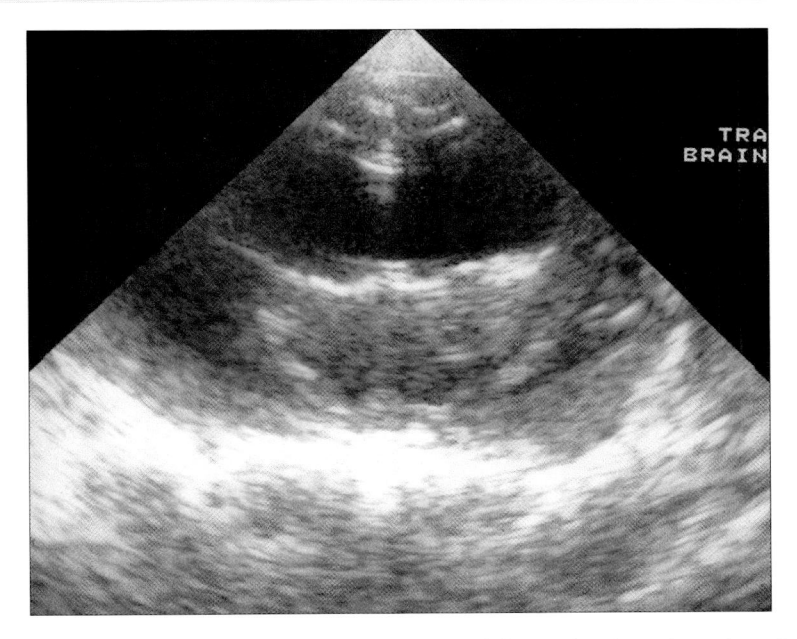

**140** A six-month-old Yorkshire terrier is presented for evaluation of ataxia, seizures, and dementia. Evaluate the sonogram of the brain performed through the fontanelle.

**141** A young adult cat is presented with an acute onset of paraplegia. There is no history of trauma. The cat has firm, areflexic pelvic limbs. There is no pulse in the femoral arteries. The digits do not bleed when pricked with a needle.
i. What is the diagnosis?
ii. What is the pathogenesis?
iii. Describe the treatment and prognosis.

# 140 & 141: Answers

**140** The lateral ventricles are enlarged and confluent. Ultrasonography performed through a fontanelle is a simple, non-invasive technique for assessing lateral ventricular size in animals suspected of having hydrocephalus. Clinical signs associated with hydrocephalus include an enlarged, domed calvarium, ventrolateral strabismus, depression, dementia, seizures, blindness, vestibular dysfunction, and ataxia. The lateral ventricles of normal dogs appear as two slit-like anechoic areas with dorsoventral height of approximately 0.15 cm. Because there is a poor correlation between ventricular size and clinical signs, the diagnosis of hydrocephalus should be based on clinical signs as well as imaging studies. If a fontanelle is not present, CT or MRI may be used to image the ventricles.

### References
Hudson JA, Simpson ST, Buxton DF, Cartee RE, Steiss JE. Ultrasonographic diagnosis of canine hydrocephalus. *Vet Radiol* 1990; 31: 50–58.
Spaulding KA, Sharp NJH. Ultrasonographic imaging of the lateral cerebral ventricles in the dog. *Vet Radiol* 1990; 31: 59–64.
Rivers WJ, Walter PA. Hydrocephalus in the dog: utility of ultrasonography as an alternate diagnostic technique. *J Am Anim Hosp Assn* 1992;28: 333–342.

**141 i.** Ischaemic neuromyopathy (iliac thrombosis, aortic embolism).
**ii.** This disorder is seen in cats with underlying cardiomyopathy. Thrombus formation occurs in the heart, with subsequent embolisation of material, which becomes lodged in the distal aorta. This usually occurs near the bifurcation, affecting the iliac arteries. Collateral circulation is impaired, probably due to release of vasoactive substances. There are pathological changes in the skeletal muscles and peripheral nerves.
**iii.** Treatment is aimed at stabilising the cat with suitable fluid therapy and cardiac medications. Medications aimed at promoting reperfusion have been recommended: acepromazine for vasodilation, heparin to inhibit coagulation, aspirin for antiplatelet activity. All these medications have potentially severe side-effects. Thrombolytic therapy has been evaluated, but it may be hazardous. Surgical removal of the thrombi has been described. The possibility of reperfusion injury must be considered (reperfusion causes hyperkalaemia and metabolic acidosis). Whatever method of treatment is selected, the prognosis is guarded. The neurological status will improve in approximately 50% of cats, but the underlying cardiac disease may be difficult to resolve and recurrences can occur.

### Reference
Pion PD, Kittleson MD. Therapy for feline aortic thromboembolism. In: Kirk RW (ed). *Current Veterinary Therapy X*. Philadelphia: Saunders, 1989: 295.

## 142–144: Questions

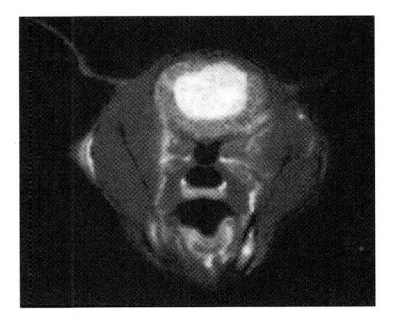

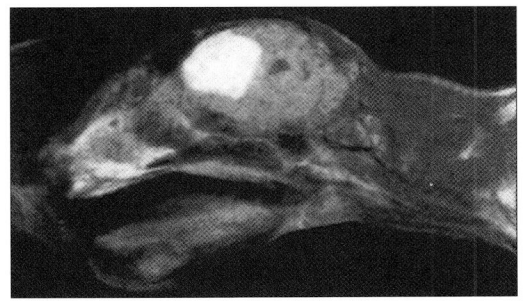

**142** You are presented with a nine-year-old domestic cat. The cat lives indoors. It has recently suffered several seizures. Physical examination is unremarkable. The neurological examination reveals reduced CP (+1) in the pelvic limbs. Routine laboratory evaluations (including bile acids) are normal.
i. Localise the lesion and give the differential diagnosis.
ii. What further tests would you perform?
iii. Interpret the findings of the MRI scan ($T_1$ plus gadolinium) of the cat. Give a realistic differential diagnosis.
iv. Based on your most likely diagnosis, what treatment options are available?
v. What is the prognosis?

**143** What anaesthetic side-effects are associated with cervical ventral decompressive surgery?

**144** A four-year-old German shepherd dog with a six-month history of seizures is presented for emergency evaluation. The owner reports that the dog has been seizing for at least 30 minutes. The dog is unconscious, panting, and salivating. There are paddling and chewing movements. What is your immediate treatment?

## 142–144: Answers

**142** i. Forebrain.
ii. Intracranial imaging (CT or MRI); CSF collection if the imaging is normal.
iii. There is a large contrast-enhancing lesion in the rostral cerebrum. It is strongly and homogenously signal-intense. It has a broad area of contact with the surface of the brain. This is probably a neoplasm, most likely a meningioma, although other tumour types are possible, for example astrocytoma.
iv. Surgical resection is indicated for many meningiomas.
v. The prognosis is reasonably good, although there is a risk of death in the immediate postoperative period, usually due to brain herniation. One study indicated that local recurrence occurs in approximately one quarter of cats that recover from surgery.

### Reference
Gallagher JG, Berg J, Knowles KE, Williams LL, Bronson RT. Prognosis after surgical excision of cerebral meningiomas in cats: 17 cases (1986–1992). *J Am Vet Med Assn* 1993; **203**: 1437–1440.

**143** Cardiac arrhythmias (bradycardia and ventricular premature contractions) were seen in 31% of dogs in one study, which was 2.5 times more frequent than in thoracolumbar disc surgery. Two of 48 dogs died following surgery.

### Reference
Stauffer J-L, Gleed RD, Short CE, Erb HN, Schlikken YH. Cardiac dysrhythmias during anesthesia for cervical decompression in the dog. *Am J Vet Res* 1988; **49**: 1143–1146.

**144** Administer diazepam (0.5–1 mg/kg, intravenously). The dog is suffering from status epilepticus. The initial goal of therapy is immediate termination of the seizure. The longer an episode of status epilepticus goes untreated, the more difficult it is to control and the greater the risk of permanent brain damage. Diazepam enters the brain quickly and usually stops status epilepticus. If the seizure does not stop within five minutes, the diazepam should be repeated. If the seizure persists after three doses, pentobarbital (3–15 mg/kg, intravenously, slowly to effect) should be administered.

An adequate airway should be secured. Intubation and ventilation may be required. An intravenous catheter should be placed and blood samples obtained for glucose and calcium concentrations. The dog's temperature should be monitored and any hyperthermia treated. Glucocorticoid adminstration has been recommended for animals with status epilepticus to treat possible cerebral oedema.

### Reference
Lane SB, Bunch SE. Medical management of recurrent seizures in dogs and cats. *J Vet Intern Med* 1990; **4**: 26–39.

## 145 & 146: Questions

**145** Regarding the dog in Q144, the seizure stops within one minute of intravenous administration of diazepam. The dog remains unresponsive. Thirty minutes later, the dog suffers another generalised motor seizure. What is your next step?

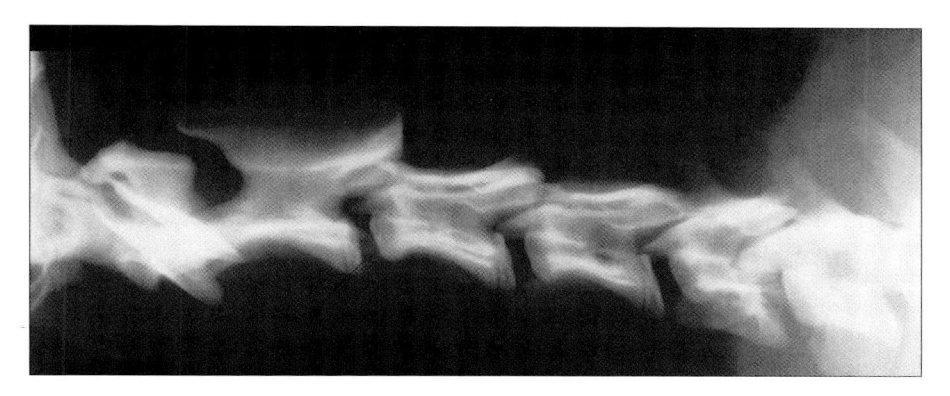

**146** A one-year-old Rottweiler is hit by a motor car. On examination one hour after the accident, the dog is recumbent and tetraparetic with feeble voluntary movement and intact spinal reflexes in all limbs. You perform a lateral radiograph of the cervical spine.
i. Evaluate the radiograph (**above**).
ii. What medical therapy would you recommend?
iii. What are the potential complications associated with medical management of this dog?

## 145 & 146: Answers

**145** Repeat the initial dose of diazepam and administer phenobarbitone (2–4 mg/kg, intramuscularly). Because diazepam is a highly lipid soluble, it is quickly redistributed, causing brain and serum concentrations to fall. Therefore, status epilepticus frequently recurs if diazepam alone is used. A longer-lasting anticonvulsant, such as phenobarbitone, should be given as needed, usually twice daily, in conjunction with diazepam. Approximately 20 minutes are needed for phenobarbitone to enter the brain and exert anticonvulsant activity, so the seizure should initially be stopped with diazepam. Once the seizures are controlled, a diagnostic evaluation should be performed to detect the cause of the seizures.

**146** i. There is a comminuted fracture of the fifth cervical vertebral body with narrowing of the C5/C6 intervertebral disc space. The vertebral canal does not appear to be substantially compromised, although myelography would be necessary to define the extent of any spinal cord compression.
ii. Methylprednisolone sodium succinate (30 mg/kg, administered intravenously as early as possible after injury) may improve the outcome of spinal cord trauma. A second dose of 15 mg/kg should be administered two hours after the initial dose, followed every six hours by a 15 mg/kg dose or, alternatively, the equivalent amount (5.4 mg/kg) infused every hour. This regimen should be continued for 24–48 hours. Cage confinement and external support of the cervicothoracic area are important to decrease movement at the fracture site. Analgesics and sedatives are also indicated.
Many vertebral fractures, especially cervical fractures, are amenable to conservative therapy. Surgery should be considered if the neurological status deteriorates, to provide decompression if there is radiographic or myelographic evidence of substantial spinal cord compression, or to provide internal fixation of very unstable fractures.
iii. A potential complication is deterioration in neurological status due to vertebral instability. Respiratory insufficiency due to paresis of the intercostal muscles is a potential life-threatening complication of severe lesions of the cervical portion of the spinal cord. Side-effects of glucocorticoid therapy in animals with spinal cord injuries include GI ulceration, immunosuppression, and disturbances of glucose and nitrogen metabolism. However, the risk of side-effects increases more in relation to duration of administration than the dose. Meticulous nursing care is important to avoid decubital ulcers and soiling with urine and faeces.

### References
Braughler JM, Hall ED. Current application of 'high-dose' steroid therapy for CNS injury. *J Neurosurg* 1985; **62**: 806–810.
Selcer RR, Bubb WJ, Walker TL. Management of vertebral column fractures in dogs and cats: 211 cases (1977–1985). *J Am Vet Med Assn* 1991; **198**: 1965–1968.

## 147–149: Questions

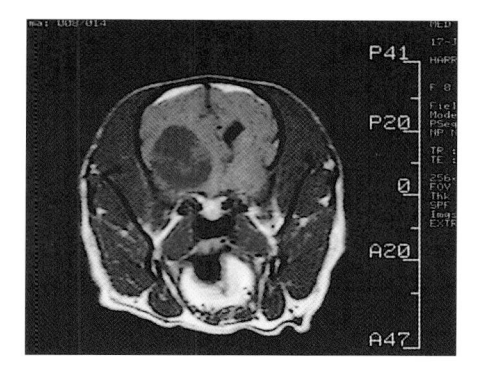

**147** These are MRI images (a–T1, b–T1 plus gadolinium, and c–T2) of a nine-year-old Miniature poodle with signs of forebrain disease. Interpret the images.

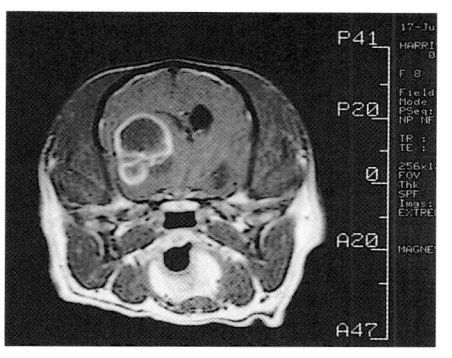

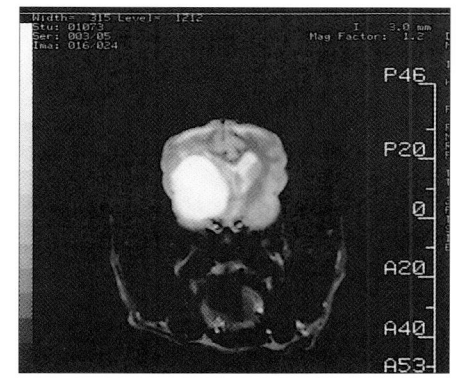

**148** What are the potential hazards of using prolonged courses of corticosteroids in dogs with spinal disorders?

**149** A previously healthy, five-year-old Dachshund has surgery (ventral slot and fenestration) for an extruded intervertebral disc at C2/C3. Which of the following is appropriate regarding analgesics in the immediate postoperative period?
a) Analgesics are contraindicated because they will encourage increased activity.
b) The side-effects of analgesics outweigh any potential benefits.
c) Analgesics should be given if and when the dog shows signs of pain.
d) Something other than the above.

## 147–149: Answers

**147** There is an abnormality in the left aspect of the cerebrum. On the T1 image the lesion is of low signal intensity, with some small areas of higher intensity traversing the lesion. The T1 plus gadolinium image shows that only the margin of the lesion is contrast-enhancing. The T2 image shows the lesion to be uniformly of high signal intensity.

This is typical of a glioma with a cystic structure. Other considerations would be cystic meningioma or inflammatory lesion, but these are far less likely.

**Reference**
Thomas WB, Wheeler SJ, Kornegay JN, Kramer R. Magnetic resonance imaging of primary brain tumors in dogs. *Vet Radiol Ultrasound*. (In press).


**148** Immunosuppression and impaired wound healing are familiar complications of corticosteroid use. This is of particular concern in neurosurgical patients.

Many dogs referred for decompressive surgery for disc herniations have been treated in the preceding days or weeks with corticosteroids. Corticosteroids relieve discomfort, but make the dog much more active, rendering it very susceptible to further herniation of disc material and subsequent development of severe neurological deficits.

Corticosteroids can cause GI bleeding in as many as 15% of neurosurgical patients, with mortality rates of up to 2%. Dexamethasone is most likely to cause these problems, but there is little evidence that this drug is of benefit in CNS injury and it is of doubtful value in experimental acute spinal cord trauma.

**Reference**
Moore RW, Withrow SJ. Gastrointestinal hemorrhage and pancreatitis associated with intervertebral disc disease in the dog. *J Am Vet Med Assn* 1982; **180**: 1443–1447.


**149** d) A procedure such as cervical spinal surgery will cause significant pain and the clinician should provide appropriate analgesia. The stress response to postoperative pain increases morbidity and slows recovery. Analgesic administration on an 'as needed' basis is not sufficient, as this ensures the dog will suffer pain, and the presence and degree of pain is often difficult to evaluate objectively. With good patient care, including the use of appropriate dosages of analgesics, postoperative pain can usually be controlled without deleterious side-effects.

**Reference**
Hansen B. Analgesics in cardiac, surgical, and intensive care patients. In: Kirk RW, Bonagura JD (eds). *Current Veterinary Therapy XI*. Philadelphia: Saunders, 1992: 82–87.

## 150–152: Questions

**150** Regarding the dog in **Q149**, which of the following is the most appropriate protocol for management of pain in the immediate postoperative period?
a) Acetylpromazine at 0.1 mg/kg, intravenously, every six hours.
b) Pentazocine at 3 mg/kg, intravenously, every six hours.
c) Oxymorphone at 0.1 mg/kg, intravenously, every six hours.
d) Meperidine at 5 mg/kg, intramuscularly, every six hours.
e) Dexamethasone at 0.1 mg/kg, intravenously, every 12 hours.

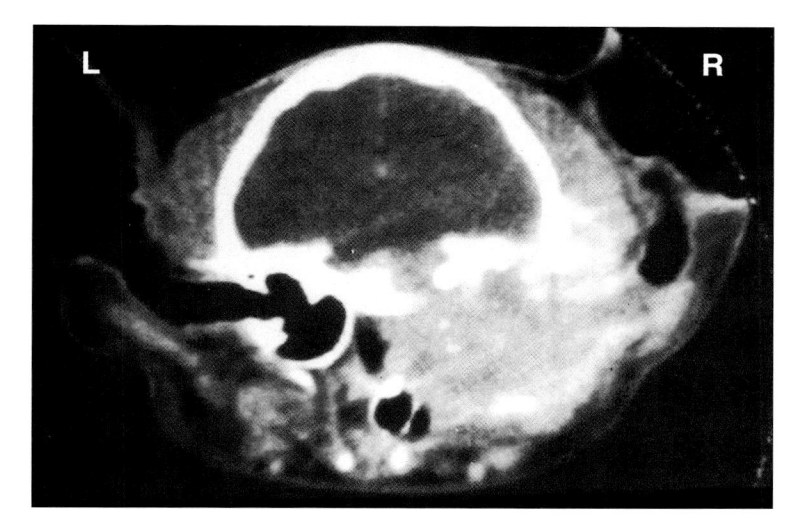

**151** The transverse CT scan is from a nine-year-old cat with a three-month duration of a head tilt to the right. What are the differential diagnoses?

**152** How do the degenerative processes that occur in the intervertebral discs vary between chondrodystrophoid and non-chondrodystrophoid breeds of dog? What clinical implications does this carry?

## 150–152: Answers

**150** c) Of those listed, oxymorphone is the best choice for moderate to severe postoperative pain. Acetylpromazine is not analgesic, although its sedative and anti-anxiety effects may be beneficial when combined with analgesics to control pain in anxious animals. Pentazocine, an opioid agonist-antagonist, is considered ineffective for most types of postoperative pain. Meperidine's use is limited by its short duration of action. Corticosteroids, such as dexamethasone, act primarily by suppressing inflammation. Their relatively poor analgesic properties and potential for severe side-effects, such as GI ulceration, make them a poor choice for postoperative pain control.

### References
Hansen B. Analgesics in cardiac, surgical, and intensive care patients. In: Kirk RW, Bonagura JD (eds). *Current Veterinary Therapy XI*. Philadelphia: Saunders, 1992: 82–87.
Sackman JE. Pain. Part II: control of pain in animals. *Compend Contin Educat Pract Vet* 1991; **13**: 181–192.

**151** Soft tissue is obliterating the right nasopharyngeal region and part of the external ear canal. There is destruction of the right tympanic bulla and part of the temporal bone. Lytic lesions of the tympanic bulla are usually neoplastic. In a cat the primary considerations are squamous cell carcinoma and ceruminous gland tumours. Diagnosis can be confirmed by examining biopsy tissue. Due to the extent of the lesion in this cat, the prognosis is poor. The histological diagnosis was squamous cell carcinoma.

**152** Two types of disc degeneration occur, and these may precede disc herniation:
• Chondroid metamorphosis occurs in chondrodystrophoid breeds in the first two years of life. As the disc degenerates it dehydrates and the nucleus pulposus is invaded by hyaline cartilage. This interferes with the shock-absorbing capacity of the disc by reducing the hydrostatic properties of its normally fluid-filled nucleus pulposus and by weakening the fibres of the annulus fibrosus. In most Dachshunds by two years of age the majority of discs have undergone chondroid metamorphosis, and many nuclei have also mineralised, changing from the former jelly-like consistency to a dry, gritty substance. Normal use often causes severe weakening of the intervertebral discs, especially at the thoracolumbar junction. This explains why the peak incidence of disc disease is between 3–6 years of age for most chondrodystrophoid breeds, termed Hansen Type I herniation or 'disc extrusion'.
• Fibroid metamorphosis occurs in non-chondrodystrophoid breeds late in life. The nucleus pulposus also dehydrates, but is invaded by fibrocartilage. This has a later onset than chondroid metamorphosis and the discs are usually normal while the dog is young and active. The nucleus pulposus does not mineralise as often as in discs with chondroid metaplasia. The disc bulges into the vertebral canal, causing a low grade myelopathy in older dogs, and is termed Hansen Type II herniation or 'disc protrusion'.

### Reference
Hansen HJ. A pathologic-anatomical study on disc degeneration in dogs. *Acta Orthop Scand* 1952; Supplement **11**.

## 153–155: Questions

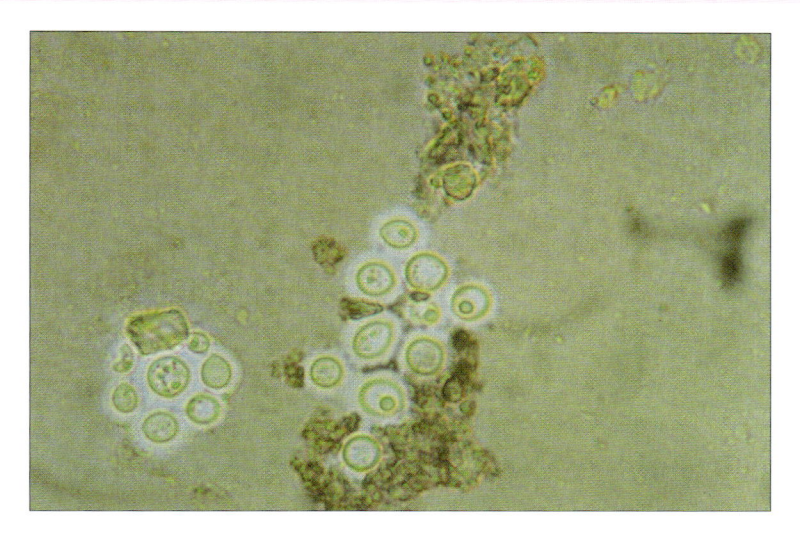

**153** You examine a four-year-old cat because of generalised seizures that began three weeks before evaluation. The owner and cat have recently moved from the southwestern United States. The cat appears slightly depressed but no other neurological deficits are detected. Cerebrospinal fluid analysis discloses a normal nucleated cell count (2 mononuclear cells per µl) and a mildly increased protein concentration (27 mg/dl; normal <25 mg/dl). An India ink preparation of the CSF is shown (**above**). What is the diagnosis and treatment?

**154** A five-year-old Golden retriever is presented with an abnormal eye. The right pupil is smaller than the left. In the right eye the third eyelid is protruded and there is ptosis of the upper lid.
i. What is this syndrome?
ii. Where could the lesion be and what could be the underlying cause?
iii. How would you try to determine the site of the lesion?
iv. You apply 10% phenylephrine to the eyes. The right pupil dilates in 20 minutes; the left eye takes 40 minutes. What does this tell you about the location of the lesion?

**155** A seven-year-old Springer spaniel is presented for an acute onset of blindness. Both pupils are dilated and unresponsive to light. Menace response and visual following are absent bilaterally. Localise the lesion.

# 153–155: Answers

**153** The cytological preparation shows multiple yeast-like organisms surrounded by a clear capsule. This finding is consistent with a diagnosis of cryptococcosis. A latex agglutination test and culture are useful in supporting a cytological diagnosis or in cases where the organism can not be identified cytologically.

Approximately 17% of cats with cryptococcosis have involvement of the nervous system. Other common sites of involvement include the upper respiratory system, skin, and eyes. In cats with cryptococcal infection of the central nervous system the inflammatory response is often mild. A careful search for the organism and a cryptococcal antigen test should be performed in any cat with central nervous system dysfunction, even if CSF analysis does not indicate inflammatory disease. Although amphotericin B in combination with flucytosine has been recommended, fluconazole (50 mg orally, twice a day) is probably the drug of choice for treating feline cryptococcosis.

**Reference**
Ackerman L. Feline cryptococcosis. *Compend Contin Educat Pract Vet* 1988: **10**: 1049–1055.

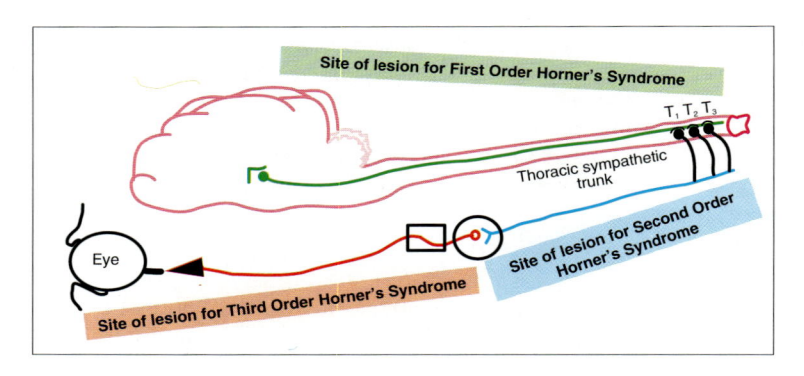

**154 i.** Horner's syndrome.
**ii.** See illustration **above** (also **A1**). Causes of Horner's syndrome: First Order – cervical and cranial thoracic spinal injuries; Second Order – brachial plexus root lesions and injuries to the soft tissues of the neck (eg, puncture, injections, iatrogenic); Third Order – middle ear lesions (otitis, neoplasia), skull fractures, retrobulbar contusions, and iatrogenic.
**iii.** Perform a full physical examination, with emphasis on the head and neck, and a full neurological examination. Consider chest radiographs.
**iv.** This indicates that this is a third order Horner's syndrome – the lesion is distal to the cranial cervical ganglion. See illustration for causes.

**155** Blindness with dilated, unresponsive pupils indicates a lesion in the eyes, optic nerves, optic chiasma, or optic tracts.

## 156–158: Questions

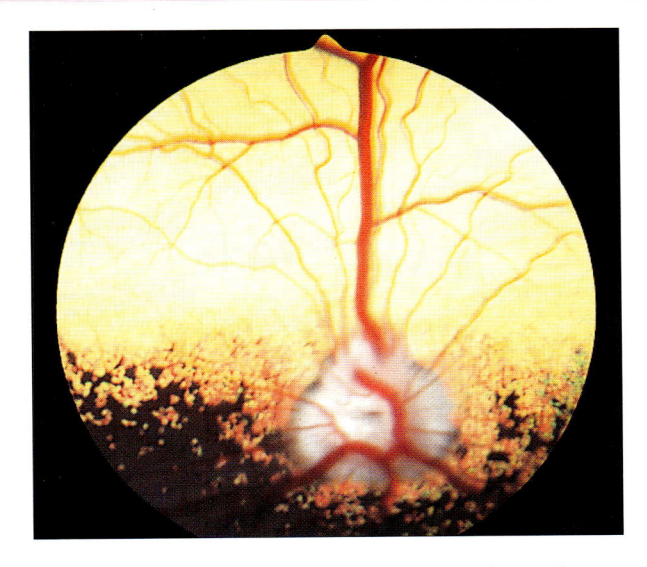

**156** Regarding the dog in **Q155**, no abnormalities are detected on examination of the cornea, anterior segment, and lens. The fundus is shown (**above**). What are your differential diagnoses and recommendations?

**157** How is potassium bromide generally used as an anticonvulsant in dogs?

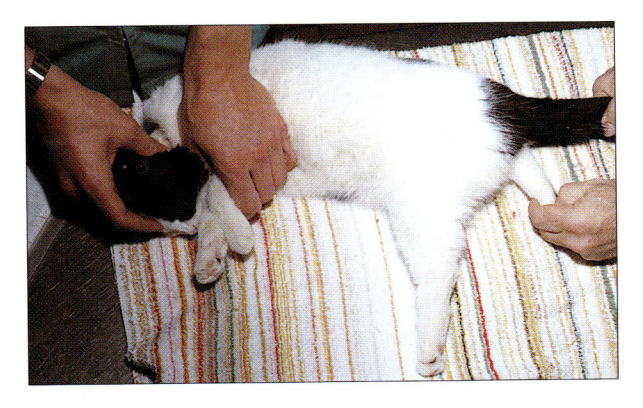

**158** What neurological finding is illustrated? What is the significance of this finding?

## 156–158: Answers

**156** The fundus appears normal. The primary diagnostic considerations for acute blindness with dilated, unresponsive pupils and a normal eye examination are optic neuritis and sudden acquired retinal degeneration (SARD). In cases of optic neuritis the fundus may appear normal, or there may be elevation and swelling of the optic disc and haemorrhage of the disc and peripapillary retina. Optic neuritis may be caused by bacterial, mycotic, protozoal, or algal infection, distemper, lymphoma, or granulomatous meningoencephalomyelitis. Many cases are idiopathic. SARD is characterised by acute, bilateral degeneration of the photoreceptors of unknown cause. Many dogs with SARD develop temporary signs of hyperadrenocorticism at about the same time as the onset of blindness. Initially, fundoscopy is normal, but after several weeks to months vascular attenuation and tapetal hyper-reflectivity develop. There is no treatment for SARD and blindness is permanent.

An electroretinogram (ERG) should be performed urgently to differentiate optic neuritis from SARD. If the ERG reveals no retinal activity, the diagnosis is SARD. If the ERG is normal, optic neuritis is likely and further diagnostic tests, including CSF analysis, are indicated in an attempt to identify the underlying cause. If an infectious agent is not identified, prednisolone (2.2 mg/kg daily) should be administered. Early treatment may result in return of vision. If no improvement is seen, the prognosis for return of vision is poor.

**Reference**
Neaderland MH. Sudden blindness. In: Kirk RW, Bonagura JD (eds). *Current Veterinary Therapy XI*. Philadelphia: Saunders, 1992: 644–647.

**157** Potassium bromide is used in dogs that do not respond to conventional anticonvulsant medication. It is generally used as an addition to phenobarbitone. It is usual to administer phenobarbitone such that the serum concentration reaches the top of the therapeutic range (10–40 µg/ml), and then to add potassium bromide if the clinical response is not satisfactory. It is sometimes possible to reduce the phenobarbitone concentration and still maintain an adequate clinical response.

**Reference**
Schwartz-Porsche D.. Management of refractory seizures. In: Kirk RW, Bonagura JD (eds). *Current Veterinary Therapy XI*. Philadelphia: Saunders, 1992: 986–991.

**158** Crossed extensor reflex. This reflex consists of extension of the limb opposite to the one in which a flexor reflex is elicited. This is an abnormal reflex in a recumbent dog or cat. The presence of a crossed extensor reflex indicates an upper motor lesion, ie. a lesion cranial to L4 for the pelvic limbs and cranial to C6 for the thoracic limbs. Other signs of UMN involvement (loss of voluntary movement, exaggerated patellar reflexes) would be expected.

# 159–161: Questions

**159** A 10-year-old cat is hospitalised for fluid therapy (lactated Ringer's solution) to treat chronic renal failure. On the third day of hospitalisation the cat appears weak, depressed, and sits with the neck flexed (**right**). Neurological examination reveals generalised weakness. Results of laboratory evaluation with reference ranges are shown in the Table. What do you recommend?

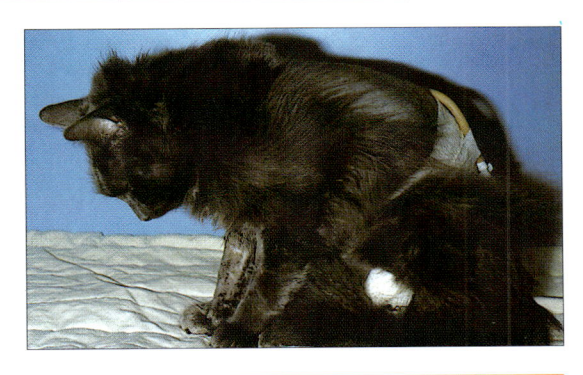

| Parameter | Result | Reference range |
|---|---|---|
| Serum urea | 20 mmol/l | 4.0–11.0 |
| Creatinine | 205 µmol/l | 40–180 |
| Sodium | 150 mmol/l | 150–165 |
| Potassium | 2.1 mmol/l | 3.7–5.8 |
| Chloride | 115 mmol/l | 112–130 |
| Glucose | 5.8 mmol/l | 3.5–6.0 |
| Total protein | 6.2 g/l | 6.0–8.2 |
| Packed cell volume | 22% | 30–45 |
| White blood cell count | 22,700/µl | 6,500–30,000 |

**160** i. In what circumstances during spinal surgery is the use of prophylactic antibiotics indicated?
ii. What antibiotics are most suitable?

**161** The illustration (**right**) shows testing of the perineal reflex.
i. What is the expected normal response?
ii. What spinal cord segments and peripheral nerve(s) does this test evaluate?

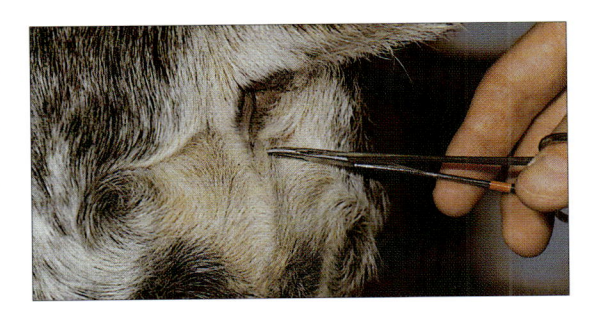

## 159–161: Answers

**159** Ventral flexion of the neck is a common manifestation of neuromuscular weakness in the cat. Common causes are hypokalaemia, hyperthyroidism, and thiamine deficiency. Less common causes include myasthenia gravis, polymyositis, polyneuropathy, hypocalcaemia, hepatic encephalopathy, and muscular dystrophy. The findings of serum potassium concentration of less than 3.0 mmol/l and muscle weakness is highly suggestive of hypokalaemic myopathy. Oral administration of potassium is the safest treatment. The serum potassium concentration should be monitored daily.

### Reference
Dow SW, LeCouteur RA, Fettman MJ, Spurgeon TL. Potassium depletion in cats: hypokalemic polymyopathy. *J Am Vet Med Assn* 1987; **191**: 1563–1568.


**160 i.** Most neurosurgical procedures are classified as clean and uncontaminated, and do not require prophylactic antibiotics unless sterility is broken or one or more of the following factors apply: skin infection or inflammation; periodontal disease; urinary infections; obesity; shock; sepsis; use of implants; Cushing's disease; long surgery (>90 mins); excessive electrocautery.
**ii.** Cephazolin (20 mg/kg intravenously) is recommended because of its good tissue penetration and broad spectrum of activity against staphylococci and other Gram-positive organisms.

Prophylactic antibiotics are used from the start of surgery to a maximum of three hours afterwards – it is at this time that bacterial contamination of tissue can be suppressed by antimicrobial therapy. There is no advantage in using intravenous antibiotics before the start of surgery, or for continuing them beyond its completion, except in concomitant diseases such as pyoderma or urinary tract infection.

### Reference
Richardson DC, Aucoin DP, DeYoung DJ, Tyczcowska KL, DeYoung BA. Pharmacokinetic disposition of cephazolin in serum and tissue during canine total hip replacement. *Vet Surg* 1992; **21**: 1–4.


**161 i.** The perineal reflex is initiated by gentle stimulation of the perineum. Normal response is contraction of the anal sphincter and flexion of the tail.
**ii.** Sensory innervation is carried by the pudendal nerve to the S1–S3 spinal cord segments. Motor innervation to the external anal sphincter is via the pudendal nerve. Flexion of the tail is mediated by the caudal nerves. Depression or absence of this reflex indicates a lesion of the sacral spinal cord segments or the pudendal nerves.

## 162–164: Questions

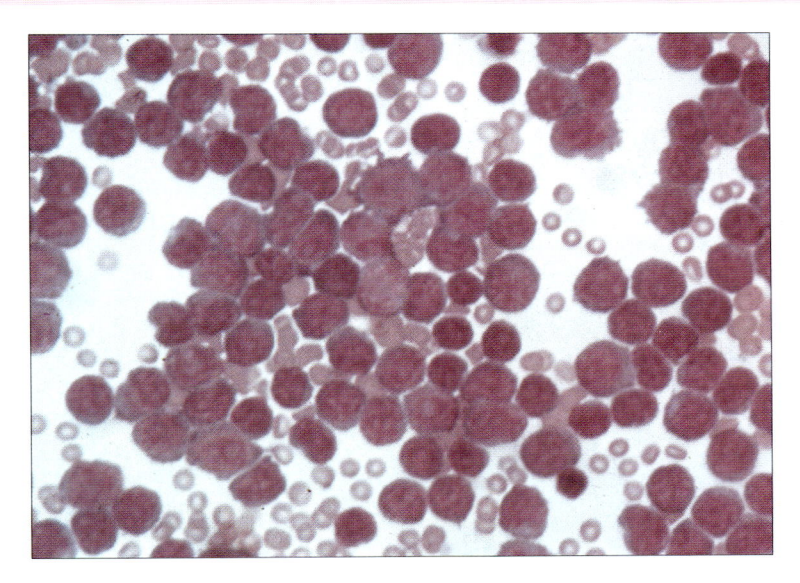

**162** A nine-year-old Dobermann is examined because of weakness of three-weeks duration. Postural reactions are decreased in all limbs (+1). Spinal reflexes and cranial nerves are normal. Prior to myelography, CSF is collected (1,745 nucleated cells/µl – normal <5 cells/µl; and 87.5 mg/dl protein – normal <25 mg/dl). The cytocentrifuge preparation of CSF is shown (**above**).
i.   What is your diagnosis?
ii.  How would you manage this case?

**163** What are the potential neurological complications of the following surgical procedures?
i.   Perineal hernia repair.
ii.  Acetabular fracture repair.
iii. Bulla osteotomy.
iv.  Thyroidectomy.
v.   Femoral fracture intramedullary pin placement.

**164** A four-year-old cat is presented with a recent onset of anorexia and ataxia. The cat is depressed with dilated pupils. Further examination causes the cat to suffer severe flexion of the spine, especially the neck, followed by a clonic seizure lasting approximately 30 seconds. What question do you ask the owner?

# 162–164: Answers

**162 i.** Lymphoma. The CSF contains large lymphoid cells with multiple nucleoli, scanty cytoplasm, and vacuolisation. Most dogs with CNS lymphoma have multicentric disease, but primary CNS lymphoma has been reported (Couto et al, 1984). Clinical signs vary depending on the area of the CNS affected, but signs of spinal cord involvement are common. Diagnosis is based on the results of blood analysis, bone marrow examination, lymph node cytology, CSF analysis, myelography, MRI or CT, and biopsy. Neoplastic cells may occasionally be found in the CSF in patients with lymphoma.

**ii.** Radiation therapy should be considered initially in animals with CNS involvement because of the rapid reduction in tumour size induced by this mode of therapy. There are several chemotherapeutic protocols available for treatment of lymphoma (Vail, 1993). Cytosine arabinoside and prednisone achieve relatively high concentrations in the CSF and have been used for the treatment of lymphoma with CNS involvement (Couto et al, 1984). Therapy often results in substantial improvement in clinical signs, although cures are rare.

### References
Couto CG, Cullen J, Pedroia V, Turrel JM. Central nervous system lymphosarcoma in the dog. *J Am Vet Med Assn* 1984; **184**: 809–813.
Vail DM. Recent advances in chemotherapy for lymphoma of dogs and cats. *Compend Contin Educat Pract Vet* 1993; **15**: 1031–1037.

**163 i.** If the method of repair is by suturing the external anal sphincter to the sacrotuberous ligament, the sciatic nerve can easily be damaged. The sciatic nerve lies close to the sacrotuberous ligament and it can be damaged by attempts to pass sutures around the ligament.

**ii.** Damage to the main trunk of the sciatic nerve as it runs dorsomedial to the acetabulum. Similar damage can occur during total hip replacement.

**iii.** Horner's syndrome, facial paralysis, and peripheral vestibular syndrome.

**iv.** Damage to the recurrent laryngeal nerve.

**v.** Retrograde pin placement can impinge on the sciatic nerve, particularly if the limb is held in abduction during placement of the pin in the proximal fragment. This can be avoided by adducting the limb during pin placement.

**164** What is the cat's diet? The clinical signs are highly suggestive of thiamine deficiency. Normal pyruvate metabolism depends on thiamine, and the neurological signs of thiamine deficiency are caused by altered carbohydrate metabolism in the brain. Common signs of thiamine deficiency in the cat are flexion of the neck, mydriasis, and seizures, but ataxia, vestibular dysfunction, and coma also occur. Thiamine deficiency may be caused by feeding improperly formulated or processed food, or diets high in fish that contains thiaminase. Anorexic cats may also become thiamine deficient. Treatment consists of administration of 5–20 mg thiamine daily for several days and correction of the diet.

## 165–167: Questions

**165** What sensory nerve in the pelvic limb is being tested?

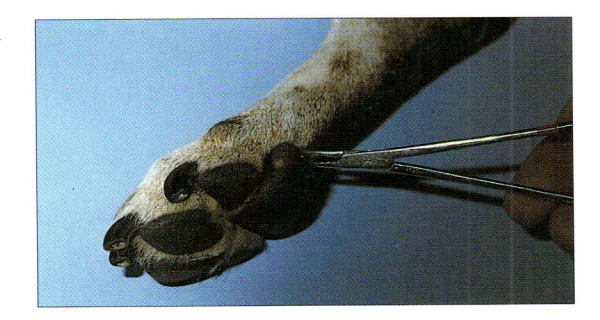

**166** A seven-year-old Labrador retriever is examined because of dyspnoea and exercise intolerance. Examination reveals inspiratory stridor but no neurological deficits. With the dog lightly anaesthetised, the larynx is examined. The arytenoid cartilages are displaced medially and ventrally and the vocal folds adduct during inspiration.
i. What is the diagnosis?
ii. How would you manage this case?

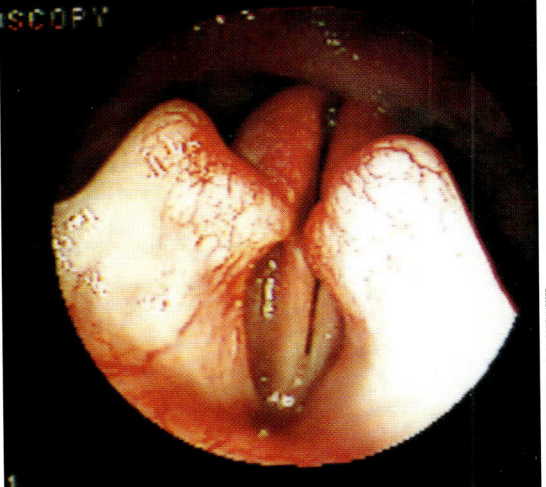

**167** Dobermanns frequently suffer from caudal cervical spondylomyelopathy ('Wobbler's syndrome') and surgical treatment is often performed. What medical problems are also seen in this breed and what tests should be performed prior to surgery?

# 165–167: Answers

**165** Pinching the plantar surface of the paw tests the tibial nerve, a branch of the sciatic nerve. The sensory function of the other branch of the sciatic nerve, the peroneal (fibular) nerve, can be tested by pinching the dorsal surface of the paw.

### Reference
Bailey CS, Kitchell RL. Cutaneous sensory testing in the dog. *J Vet Internal Med* 1987; **1**: 128–135.

**166 i.** Laryngeal paralysis. The laryngeal muscles are innervated by branches of the vagus nerve (cranial nerve X) and the internal branch of the accessory nerve (cranial nerve XI). With denervation of the laryngeal muscles, the vocal folds and arytenoid cartilages do not abduct fully during inspiration. This results in upper airway obstruction, exercise intolerance, laryngeal stridor, and dyspnoea. A hoarse bark may also be noticed. Acquired laryngeal paralysis is seen most commonly in middle-aged to older, large breed dogs. The underlying cause is often not identified. Although signs of a diffuse polyneuropathy are often not evident on neurological examination, electrodiagnostic examination indicates a generalised, subclinical polyneuropathy in some dogs with laryngeal paralysis.

**ii.** An electromyogram and nerve conduction studies would be useful to rule out a subclinical polyneuropathy. Causes of polyneuropathy include endocrinopathies (hypothyroidism, hyperinsulinism, diabetes mellitus), toxicities (heavy metals, organophosphates), paraneoplastic neuropathies, inflammatory neuropathies, and inherited neuropathies. If a treatable cause of the neuropathy is not identified, surgical therapy may be necessary to control signs of airway obstruction.

### References
Braund KG, Steinberg HS. Shores A *et al.* Laryngeal paralysis in immature and mature dogs as one sign of a more diffuse polyneuropathy. *J Am Vet Med Assn* 1989; **194**: 1735–1740.

Gaber CE, Amis TC, LeCouteur RA. Laryngeal paralysis in dogs: a review of 23 cases. *J Am Vet Med Assn* 1985; **186**: 377–380.

**167** Dobermanns are predisposed to hypothyroidism. They should be screened by assessing the T4 or by the TSH stimulation test.

Bleeding disorders. It has been estimated that 16% of Dobermanns in the USA have a bleeding tendency related to Von Willebrand's disease. The easiest way to test an animal's Von Willebrand status is to perform a standardised bleeding time test (buccal mucosa bleeding time or cuticle bleeding time).

Cardiomyopathy is seen in many large and giant breed dogs, and is usually fatal within six months of diagnosis. Even a subtle arrhythmia should not be discounted, and an ECG and echocardiogram should be performed as indicated.

### Reference
Wheeler SJ, Sharp NJH. *Small Animal Spinal Disorders*. London: Mosby-Wolfe, 1994: 139.

# 168–171: Questions

**168** What is the name of the test illustrated (**right**)? Is this a clinically useful test in the dog?

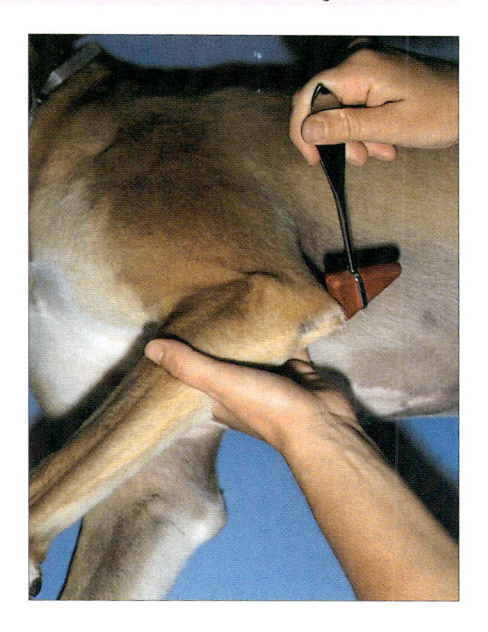

**169** How would you confirm a diagnosis of myasthenia gravis (MG)? What is the basis of the tests?

**170** You are presented with a cat that has suffered from severe flea infestation for several years. It wears a flea collar. The owners applied some insecticide originally prescribed for their dog, then noticed the instructions stated that it should not be used in cats. What clinical signs would you expect to develop and how would you counter them?

**171** Regarding hepatotoxicity caused by anticonvulsant medication, which of the following statements is *true*?
a) Increased serum alkaline phosphatase (AP) indicates liver damage.
b) Hepatotoxicity caused by chronic administration of phenobarbitone is irreversible.
c) Laboratory findings suggestive of hepatoxicity include rising serum concentrations of phenobarbitone despite a constant oral dose, proportionally larger increases in alanine aminotransferase (ALT) activity compared with alkaline phosphatase activity, and increased serum bile acids.
d) The risk of hepatoxicity is not related to the serum concentration of phenobarbitone.

## 168–171: Answers

**168** The triceps reflex is elicited by tapping the tendon of the triceps muscle. This relex is often absent in normal animals and thus is difficult to interpret.

**169** Edrophonium response test ('Tensilon test'). The animal is exercised to its limit and the time taken to collapse noted. Edrophonium hydrochloride is then given intravenously. Most animals with MG respond dramatically by rising promptly and exercising normally for several minutes. Edrophonium hydrochloride is a short acting anticholinesterase agent. By antagonising cholinesterase it potentiates the activity of acetylcholine (ACh) at the neuromuscular junction, thus increasing strength in animals where ACh activity is reduced (as in MG). Also, serum can be evaluated for antibodies to ACh receptors. Acquired MG is an immune-mediated disease and circulating antibodies to the ACh receptor are found in most patients.

**Reference**
Wheeler SJ. Disorders of the neuromuscular junction. *Progress in Vet Neurol* 1991; **2**: 129–135.

**170** Organophosphorous (OP) and carbamate insecticides interfere with acetylcholinesterase, the enzyme that inactivates acetylcholine in synapses. Cats are particularly susceptible to these agents. The clinical signs of toxicity are manifested as parasympathetic nervous system overstimulation and neuromuscular dysfunction. Animals have a stiff, rigid gait, with muscle tremors and fasciculations. Treatment includes reducing further absorption by removing the flea collar and bathing. Atropine is used to counteract the parasympathetic signs. Pralidoxime hydrochloride releases the acetylcholinesterase from the OP compound and is indicated in OP toxicity but not in carbamate toxicity.

**Reference**
Wheeler SJ. Disorders of the neuromuscular junction. *Progress in Vet Neurol* 1991; **2**: 129–135.

**171** c) Dogs receiving primidone or phenobarbitone will have moderate increases in AP and inconsistent elevations in ALT without serious abnormalities in liver function. Severe hepatic injury occasionally occurs and may be more likely if serum concentrations of phenobarbitone exceed 35 μg/ml. If the offending drug is withdrawn early enough, the damge is reversable. Because of its minimal effect on the liver, bromide is the recommended anticonvulsant for dogs with serious hepatic disease.

**References**
Bunch SE, Baldwin BH. Hornbuckle WE, Tennant BC. Compromised hepatic function in dogs treated with anticonvulsant drugs. *J Am Vet Med Assn* 1984; **184**: 444–448.
Dayrell-Hart B, Steinberg SA, Vanwinkle TJ, Farnbach GC. Hepatoxicity of phenobarbitone in dogs: 18 cases (1985–1989). *J Am Vet Med Assn* 1991; **199**: 1060–1066.

# 172 & 173 Questions

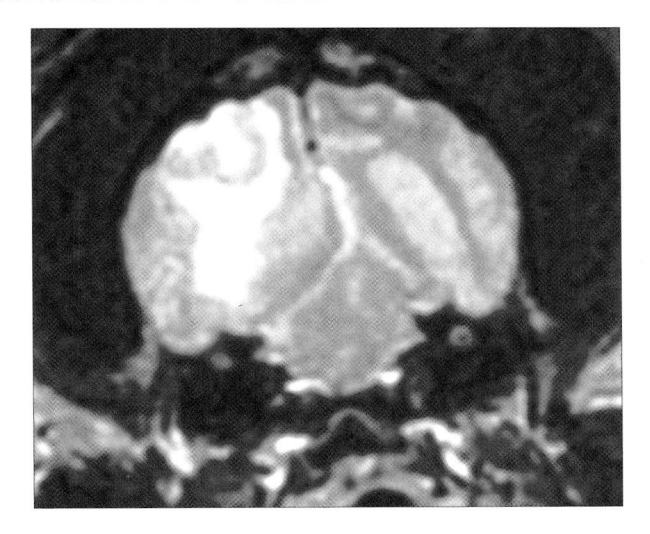

**172** A 10-year-old, mixed-breed dog undergoes general anaesthesia for MRI because of suspected intracranial neoplasia. A transverse T2-weighted image is shown. During recovery from anaesthesia the dog develops dilation of the left pupil, followed by extensor posturing, apnoea, bradycardia, and cardiac arrest.
i. What caused the dog's death?
ii. What anaesthetic protocol would you recommend to try and avoid this?

**173** A one-year-old male Dobermann is examined because of episodic collapse. The attacks are most common when the dog is eating. The owner says the dog suddenly becomes weak then collapses, during which time it remains conscious but unable to move. The episode lasts approximately 30 seconds, then the dog behaves normally. No abnormalities are detected on physical and neurological examination.
i. What is the most likely diagnosis?
ii. What treatment do you recommend?

# 172 & 173: Answers

**172 i.** These clinical signs are typical of caudal tentorial herniation with compression of the brainstem. The MRI shows a lesion of mixed intensity located in the dorsal aspect of the left cerebral hemisphere. Adjacent to this lesion there is increased intensity of the white matter typical of vasogenic oedema. The medial aspect of the left cerebral hemisphere is displaced medially and ventrally resulting in compression of the midbrain (caudal tentorial herniation), which is the likely cause of cardiorespiratory arrest.

**ii.** Impending brain shift due to increased intracranial pressure can be compounded by anaesthesia. Anaesthetic management of dogs suspected of having an intracranial mass has been reviewed by Shores (1985) and Cornick (1992). Pretreatment with glucocorticoids and mannitol are beneficial. Inhalation anaesthetics (especially halothane), ketamine, and respiratory acidosis increase intracranial pressure by causing increased cerebral blood flow. Of the available inhalation anaesthetics, isoflurane has the least effect on intracranial pressure. Premedication with diazepam, induction with a short-acting barbituate, and maintenance with isoflurane in oxygen would be appropriate. A combination of injectable anaesthetics, such as fentanyl and droperidol, would be a good alternative. Ventilation should be controlled to achieve a $PaCO_2$ of 25–30 mmHg. Judicious administration of fluids and maintenance of normal arterial blood pressure are also important.

### References
Cornick JL. Anesthetic management of patients with neurological abnormalities. *Compend Contin Educat Pract Vet* 1992; **14**: 163–172.
Kornegay JN, Oliver JE, Gorgacz EJ. Clinicopathologic features of brain herniation in animals. *J Am Vet Med Assn* 1983; **182**:1111–1116.
Shores A. Neuroanesthesia. *Vet Surg* 1985; **14**: 257–263.

**173** These episodes are typical of narcolepsy-cataplexy in dogs. The most common sign of narcolepsy in dogs is cataplexy – sudden episodes of flaccid paralysis, usually brought on by excitement such as feeding or play. In contrast to seizures, cataplectic attacks are not characterised by excessive muscle activity, incontinence, or salivation. Other manifestations of narcolepsy in dogs are excessive daytime sleepiness and disrupted night-time sleep. Narcolepsy appears to be caused by impaired sleep-wake regulation associated with abnormal neurotransmitter activity in the brain. Breeding experiments indicate narcolepsy is inherited as an autosomal recessive gene in Dobermanns and Labrador retrievers. Many other breeds may be affected.

Diagnosis is usually based on the typical history. Electroencephalographic monitoring during an attack, or inducing cataplectic episodes by drug administration, such as physostigmine, may be useful in some cases. Treatment with imipramine (0.4–1.0 mg/kg, 3 times a day) or methylphenedate (0.25 mg/kg, 3 times a day) often leads to substantial improvement.

### References
Baker TL, Mitler MM, Foutz AS, Dement WC. Diagnosis and treatment of narcolepsy in animals. In: Kirk RW (ed). *Current Veterinary Therapy VIII*. Philadelphia: Saunders, 1983; 755–759.
Katherman AE. A comparative review of canine and human narcolepsy. *Compend Contin Educat Pract Vet* 1980; **11**:818–822.

## 174–176: Questions

**174** What contrast media are suitable for myelography in dogs and cats?

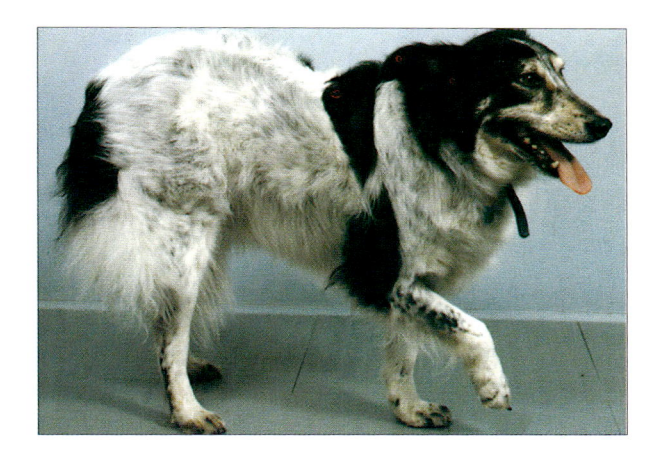

**175** This two-year-old Border collie (**above**) was involved in a road traffic accident four weeks previously. The dog initially dragged the limb, but more recently has been carrying it in the position shown here. Orthopaedic examination is normal. Neurological examination of the limb reveals an intact withdrawal reflex, although the carpus does not flex. The biceps, triceps, and extensor carpi radialis reflexes are all absent. There is severe atrophy of the triceps muscle and all muscles distal to the elbow.
i.   What is the diagnosis?
ii.  What other neurological deficits may be present? Account for these.
iii. What is the prognosis?

**176** A four-month-old West Highland white terrier is presented with a seven-week duration of progressive paraparesis. On neurological examination there is paraparesis with weak spinal reflexes (+1) in the pelvic limbs. The thoracic limbs are hypermetric and there is an intention tremor of the head.
i.   What is the neuroanatomical diagnosis?
ii.  What is the most likely diagnosis?
iii. What diagnostic tests would you perform?

## 174–176: Answers

**174** The agent must be a water-soluble, non-ionic contrast medium – iohexol (Omnipaque®, Nycomed) and iopamidol are the most often used. Metrizamide was the first of these agents to become available, but has now been superseded. The routinely used intravenous agents must not be administered as they are extremely irritant to nervous tissue and will lead to marked neurological disturbances or death.

**175** i. Brachial plexus root avulsion. (This is not 'radial paralysis', which is a very rare condition in the dog. The neurological damage is more widespread than is seen with isolated radial nerve lesions.)
ii. Horner's syndrome – the sympathetic nerve supply to the eye leaves the spinal cord in the cranial thoracic spinal nerves, some of which (T1 and T2) supply the brachial plexus. The cutaneous trunci ('panniculus') reflex may also be absent. The efferent arm of this reflex is the lateral thoracic nerve, which arises from the C8 and T1 spinal nerves. One or both of these signs is present in approximately 70% of dogs with brachial plexus root avulsion.
iii. Poor. Some improvement may occur over the first week or so after the injury, but after that recovery is unlikely.

### Reference
Wheeler SJ, Clayton Jones DG, Wright JA. The diagnosis of brachial plexus disorders in dogs: a review of twenty two cases. *J Small Anim Pract* 1986; **27**: 147–152.

**176** i. Multifocal. The paraparesis with decreased spinal reflexes indicates a lesion of the LMNs of the pelvic limbs (L4–S2 spinal cord segments or peripheral nerves). The intention tremor and thoracic limb hypermetria indicate a cerebellar lesion.
ii. Progressive multifocal signs in a young pure-bred dog are compatible with an inherited degenerative disease. Globoid cell leukodystrophy, a hereditary demyelinating disease, has been reported in West Highland white terriers. Clinical signs usually develop by the time affected dogs are several months old and initially consist of cerebellar signs or paraparesis. The disease progresses to cause abnormal behaviour, blindness, and death. Other differential diagnoses include encephalomyelitis (canine distemper virus) and toxicity (lead).
iii. Encephalitis and lead poisoning could be detected by CSF analysis and blood lead evaluation, respectively. CSF from dogs with globoid cell leukodystrophy may have increased protein and typical globoid macrophages. Peripheral nerve biopsy from affected dogs may be diagnostic for globoid cell leukodystrophy (Vicini *et al*, 1988). Definitive diagnosis is often made at necropsy, as there is no effective treatment.

### References
Fletcher TF, Kurtz HJ. Globoid cell leukodystrophy, Krabbe's disease. Animal model: globoid cell leukodystrophy in the dog. *Am J Pathol* 1972; **66**: 375–378.
Vicini DS, Wheaton LG, Zachary JF. Peripheral nerve biopsy for diagnosis of globoid cell leukodystrophy in a dog. *J Am Vet Med Assn* 1988; **192**: 1087–1090.

# 177–179: Questions

**177** This is a gross necropsy specimen from a dog. The left side of the brain is shown on the left of the figure.
i. Describe the abnormality.
ii. What neurological deficits would you expect from this lesion?

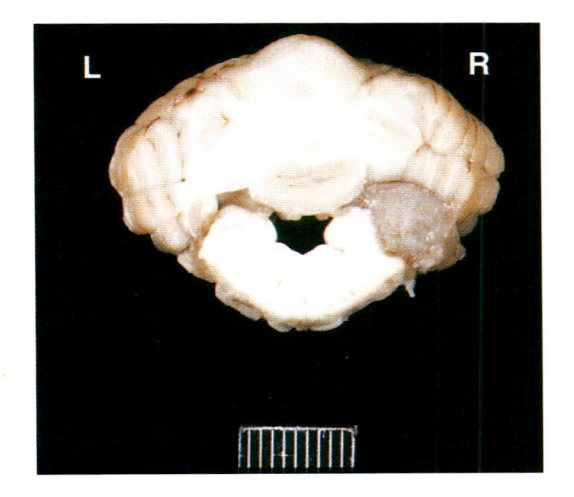

**178** Which of the following statements regarding bromide administration for epilepsy is *false*?
i. The half-life is approximately 16.5 hours and the time to reach steady-state kinetics is 8–12 days.
ii. Bromide is not appropriate for treatment of epilepsy in dogs.
iii. Side-effects include lethargy, ataxia, polyuria, and polydipsia.
iv. Bromide is excreted primarily by the kidneys.
v. The dose is 20 mg/kg/day.

**179** A two-year-old Chow Chow is presented with a 48-hour duration of paraplegia. The owner does not feel the dog could have been exposed to trauma or toxins. Examination shows absent postural reactions with intact spinal reflexes in the pelvic limbs. The menace response is absent bilaterally and the pupils are dilated and unresponsive to light. The remainder of the cranial nerves and the thoracic limbs are normal. What is the neuroanatomical diagnosis?

## 177–179: Answers

**177 i.** This is a transverse section of the cerebellum and medulla oblongata. There is a light brown mass located in the area of the right lateral aperture of the fourth ventricle. This mass is compressing the right cerebellar hemisphere and the right side of the medulla in the area of the caudal cerebellar peduncle. Choroid plexus papilloma or meningioma is most likely, although other neoplasms or granuloma are also possible.
**ii.** Right hemiparesis, ataxia, head tilt to the left, and horizontal, spontaneous nystagmus with the fast phase to the right would be the most likely signs. Compression of descending UMNs in the right side of the brainstem would cause a right hemiparesis. Lesions in the area of the caudal cerebellar peduncle usually produce a paradoxical vestibular syndrome, which is characterised by contralateral vestibular signs. Vestibular function is determined by the relative firing rates of neurons in the left and right vestibular nuclei. Neurons in the flocculus of the cerebellum travel through the caudal cerebellar peduncle and normally inhibit the ipsilateral vestibular nuclei. Loss of this inhibition by a lesion in the flocculus or caudal cerebellar peduncle results in increased firing of neurons in the ipsilateral vestibular nuclei. Increased activity of the right vestibular nuclei causes the same signs as decreased firing of the left vestibular nuclei – in other words, left vestibular signs.

### Reference
Adamo PF, Clinkscales JA. Cerebellar meningioma with paradoxical vestibular signs. *Progress Vet Neurol* 1991; 2: 137–142.

**178 i.** Actually, the elimination half-life of bromide in dogs ranges from 23–68 days and steady-state concentration is reached in 4–6 months.

### Reference
Trepainier LA. Pharmacokinetics and clinical use of bromide. *Proceedings 11th American College of Veterinary Medicine Forum.* Washington DC, 1993: 878–880.

**179** Results of the neurological examination indicate a multifocal syndrome. The paraplegia with intact spinal reflexes is caused by a lesion of the T3–L3 spinal cord segments. Blindness with absent pupillary light reflexes suggests an optic chiasma, bilateral retinal, optic nerve, or optic tract lesion.

# 180–182: Questions

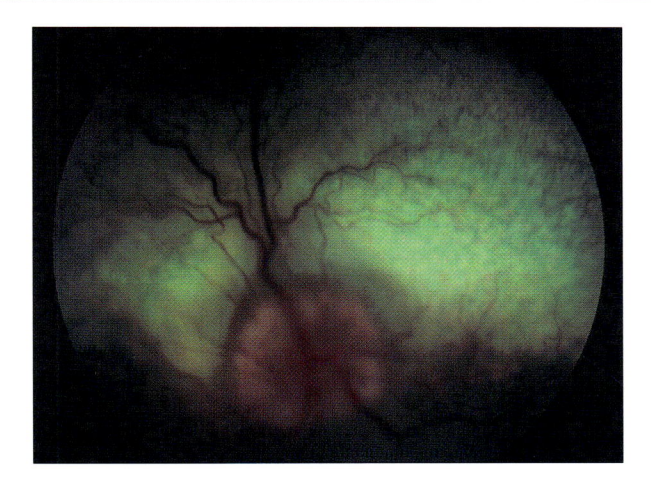

**180** The retina of the dog in **Q179** is illustrated.
i. What are the distinguishing ophthalmoscopic features?
ii. What are the differential diagnoses?

**181** A litter of 12-day-old Weimeraner puppies is presented for neurological evaluation. Three of the puppies have a generalised tremor that manifests as a rocking-type movement, most obvious in the pelvic limbs. The tremor is more severe when the puppies attempt to move and is absent during sleep. The other two puppies in the litter are normal. The bitch is healthy and the owner knows of no exposure to toxins. What do you tell the owner?

**182** An 18-month-old male Golden retriever is presented with a chronic, progressive course of generalised weakness. On examination the dog has a stilted gait, generalised muscle atrophy, and intact spinal reflexes. When supported, proprioceptive positioning is normal. No signs of pain are noticed on palpation and manipulation of the spine or major muscle groups.
i. Localise the lesion.
ii. What are the differential diagnoses?
iii. What diagnostic tests do you recommend?

## 180–182: Answers

**180** The optic disc is swollen and oedematous and the vessels are congested. These findings are consistent with optic neuritis. Acute papilloedema caused by increased intracranial pressure appears similar, but does not affect vision or pupillary light reflexes.
ii  Multifocal neurological lesions and optic neuritis strongly suggest inflammatory disease. Differential diagnoses include canine distemper, granulomatous meningoencephalitis, and fungal, protozoal, or rickettsial diseases. CSF analysis and testing for infectious diseases are indicated.

**181** Considering the age of onset and that several puppies are affected, a congenital disorder is most likely. Cerebellar malformation is possible, but tremor due to cerebellar disease is most prominent in the head. Congenital hypomyelination or dysmyelination of the central nervous system causes the type of tremor seen in these puppies. Several breeds have been affected, including Weimaraners, Springer spaniels, Samoyeds, Chow Chows, and Bernese mountain dogs. Although there is no treatment, clinical signs resolve spontaneously in Weimeraners and Chow Chows by one year of age, coincident with further myelination.

### Reference
Duncan ID. Abnormalities of myelination of the central nervous system associated with congenital tremor. *J Vet Intern Med* 1987; **1**: 10–23.

**182** i. Generalised weakness and muscle atrophy with intact proprioception and spinal reflexes is consistent with generalised muscle disease. Peripheral neuropathies can also cause generalised weakness and muscle atrophy, but usually affect proprioception and spinal cord reflexes.
ii.  Causes of generalised myopathies in dogs include myositis (*Toxoplasma gondii*, *Neospora caninum*, idiopathic polymyositis), endocrinopathies (hyperadrenocorticism, hypothyroidism), and inherited muscular dystrophy. Canine X-linked muscular dystrophy has been reported in Golden retrievers, Samoyeds, Rottweilers, and Belgian shepherd dogs. Clinical signs in Golden retrievers are noted as early as six weeks of age and include small stature, progressive weakness, pharyngeal dysfunction, muscle atrophy, and a stilted gait.
iii.  Serum creatine kinase activity is often elevated with muscular dystrophy and polymyositis. Electromyography may reveal complex repetitive discharges in many types of myopathies. Definitive diagnosis requires examination of a skeletal muscle biopsy by a pathologist familiar with techniques used in the diagnosis of muscle disorders. Before performing the biopsy, the pathologist should be consulted to provide information on obtaining and handling the sample.

### Reference
Kornegay JN. The X-linked muscular dystrophies. In: Kirk RW, Bonagura JD (eds). *Current Veterinary Therapy XI*. Philadelphia: Saunders, 1992; 1042–1047.

## 183 & 184: Questions

**183** A four-year-old Jack Russell terrier was struck by a motor car and suffered epistaxis and a fracture of the frontal bone overlying the left frontal sinus. No treatment was required and within 24 hours the dog appeared normal. Now, one week after the accident, the dog is presented for re-evaluation. Since the initial injury, the owner has observed a slight, clear nasal discharge from the left nostril. Twenty four hours ago the dog became lethargic and very painful. Examination reveals a depressed dog that is reluctant to walk and resists turning of the neck. The rectal temperature is 40°C (104°F). You are concerned that the dog has bacterial meningitis due to the skull fracture and a tear in the dura mater allowing CSF to leak into the nasal passage. Which of the following would be an appropriate antibiotic to administer while awaiting CSF analysis?
a) Cephalexin.
b) Gentamicin.
c) Tetracycline.
d) Ampicillin.

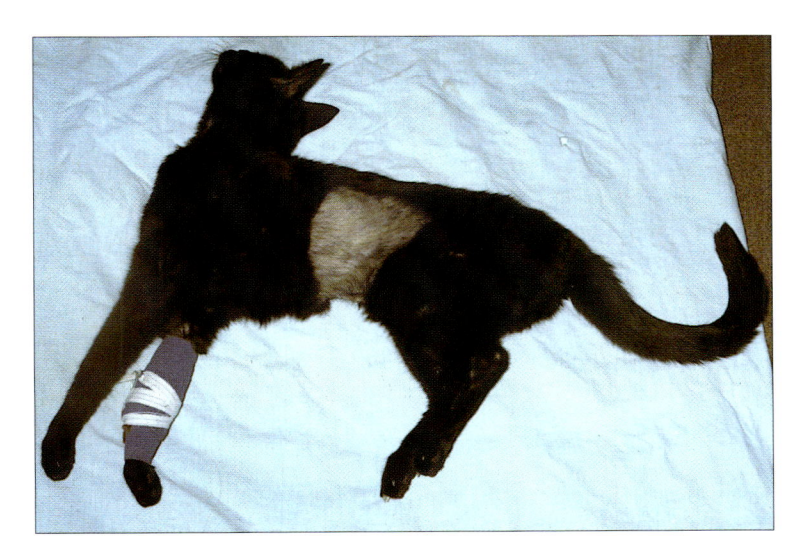

**184** A three-year-old, castrated, male domestic shorthaired cat is examined because of a two-week duration of ataxia and hypermetria progressing to the posture shown (**above**). The cat is alert, responsive, and has normal pupillary function. What is the neuroanatomical diagnosis?

# 183 & 184: Answers

**183** The primary goal of treatment of bacterial meningitis is elimination of the causative organism from the nervous system as soon as possible, before permanent damage occurs. There are several considerations in determining the choice of antibiotic. Bactericidal therapy is clearly superior to bacteriostatic therapy. Normally, the blood-CSF barrier is resistant to the passage of many antibiotics into the CSF. However, meningeal inflammation results in a marked increase in the ability of many antibiotics to cross the blood-CSF barrier.

*Staphylococcus* spp. are the most common cause of bacterial meningitis in dogs. Other organisms include *Streptococcus* spp., *Pasturella* spp., *Escherichia coli*, *Proteus* spp., *Pseudomonas* spp., and anaerobes. Ideally, the choice of therapy should be based on culture of CSF and sensitivity testing, but antibiotics should not be withheld while awaiting laboratory confirmation of a suspected case of bacterial meningitis. Initial therapy is based on the assumption that staphylococcal organisms are responsible. Intravenous administration of ampicillin (15 mg/kg, every six hours) or penicillin G (10,000–20,000 iu/kg, every 4–6 hours) should be instituted. Chloramphenicol achieves high concentrations in the CSF, but has the disadvantage of being bacteriostatic. Tetracycline is also bacteriostatic. First generation cephalosporins and aminoglycosides cross the blood-CSF barrier poorly, even in the presence of inflammation. Enrofloxacin or cefotaximine should be considered for Gram-negative meningitis. Trimethoprim/sulphonamide combinations also achieve good concentrations in the CSF.

Treatment should be continued for at least 10 days after the resolution of clinical signs. Anti-epileptic drugs and treatment for increased intracranial pressure may be necessary in some cases of meningitis. The use of glucocorticoids is controversial. The prognosis is good for mild cases given prompt therapy. Persistent neurological deficits may necessitate euthanasia in severe cases.

## References
Fenner WR. Bacterial infections of the central nervous system. In: Greene CE (ed). *Infectious Diseases of the Dog and Cat*. Philadelphia: Saunders, 1990:184–196.
Oliver JE, Lorenz MD. *Handbook of Veterinary Neurology*, 2nd ed. Philadelphia: Saunders, 1993; 105–110.

**184** This posture, characterised by opisthotonus, extension of the thoracic limbs, and flexion of the hips, has been termed decerebellate rigidity and is seen with lesions of the cerebellum. In some cases extension of the pelvic limbs can also occur. Decerebrate posturing, which occurs with severe lesions of the brainstem or cerebrum, has a similar appearance, but is less likely because the cat is alert and has normal pupillary function. The history of ataxia and hypermetria can also be explained by a cerebellar lesion.

## Reference
Holliday TA. Clinical signs of acute and chronic lesions of the cerebellum. *Vet Science Communicat* 1980; 3: 259–278.

## 185–187: Questions

**185** Regarding the cat in **Q184**, laboratory abnormalities consist of a mature neutrophilia (18,400 neutrophils per μl) and hyperglobulinemia (7.4 g/dl). Tests for FeLV and FIV were negative. A feline coronavirus titre is weakly positive at 1:200. What is the most likely diagnosis and how could this be confirmed?

**186** Upon performing a complete neurological examination on this dog, you notice the menace response is absent on the left. Postural reactions are normal. Does the dog have a visual field deficit?

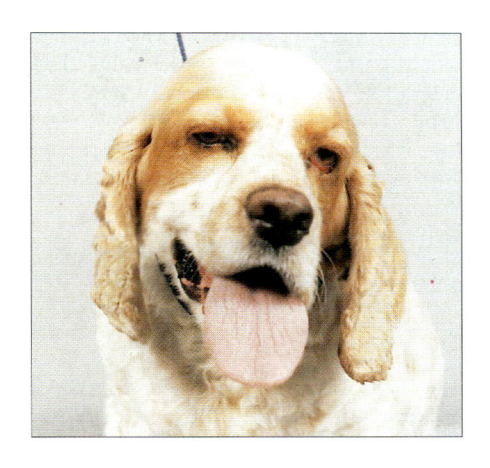

**187** A four-year-old Pekingese is presented paraplegic, of four-days duration. The dog has no deep pain sensation in the pelvic limbs. Myelography reveals a poorly-defined extradural compression in the thoracolumbar region. A dorsal laminectomy is performed. This reveals no compressive lesion, but the cord is darkly discoloured. You perform a durotomy (**above**):
i. What does this finding indicate?
ii. What is the mechanism of this process?
iii. What clinical signs may develop?
iv. What action is appropriate?

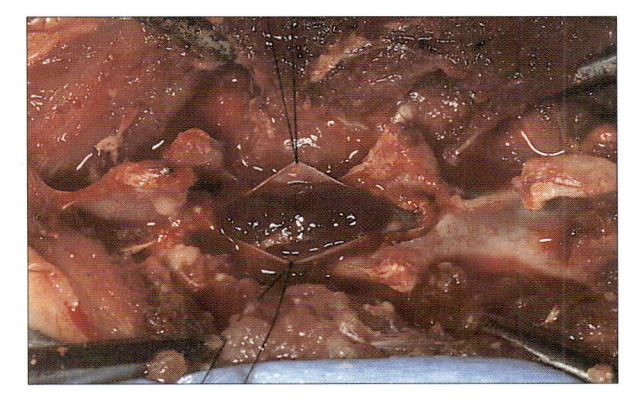

## 185–187: Answers

**185** Progressive brainstem or cerebellar signs in a cat with hyperglobulinaemia is suggestive of feline infectious peritonitis (FIP), especially the dry form. Other considerations include mycotic diseases, toxoplasmosis, rabies, and lymphoma. Low coronavirus titres are not uncommon in cats with FIP because soluble antibodies may conjugate with immune complexes and not be detected by diagnostic tests. Hydrocephalus, detectable by MRI or CT, and neutrophilic pleocytosis with increased protein on CSF evaluation are suggestive, but not diagnostic, of FIP. Imaging studies and CSF analysis would be indicated to exclude other disorders, although collection of CSF may cause deterioration in the neurological status. Definitive diagnosis requires histological examination of affected organs. Biopsy of the liver or kidney may be a useful *ante-mortem* test. The prognosis for cats with FIP and neurological involvement is grim, although corticosteroids may offer temporary improvement.

### References
Kline KL, Joseph RJ, Averill DA. Feline infectious peritonitis with neurological involvement: clinical and pathological findings in 24 cats. *J Am Anim Hosp Assn* 1994; **30**: 111–118.
Kornegay JN. Feline neurology. *Compend Contin Educat Pract Vet* 1981; **3**: 203–210.

**186** Probably not. The absent menace response is due to facial paralysis. The efferent (motor) portion of the menace response is blinking of the eye, which is mediated by the facial nerve. The dog has a head tilt to the left and drooping of the left lip. This indicates dysfunction of the left facial nerve (cranial nerve VII) and the vestibular portion of cranial nerve VIII, most likely due to a lesion of the left middle/inner ear. The visual pathway could be further evaluated by performing a visual placing test while covering the right eye.

**187** i. The dog has developed progressive myelomalacia ('the ascending syndrome').
ii. The disc material usually spreads along the epidural space for some distance, often completely encircling the dura mater. Extensive epidural and subarachnoid haemorrhage occurs, together with epidural fat necrosis, and arterial and venous thrombosis. Total or subtotal necrosis of the spinal cord can extend from the cranial thoracic to the sacral spinal cord segments.
iii. Profound depression, hyperaesthesia, and toxaemia are seen, usually developing several days after the dog becomes paralysed. There is progressive loss of pelvic limb reflexes and the level of the cutaneous trunci ('panniculus') reflex cut-off moves cranially.
iv. Euthanasia should be performed on humane grounds as affected patients will die within a few days.

### References
Davies JV, Sharp NJH. A comparison of conservative treatment and fenestration for thoracolumbar disc disease in the dog. *J Small Anim Pract* 1983; **24**: 721–729.
Griffiths IR. The extensive myelopathy of intervertebral disc protrusion in dogs ('the ascending syndrome'). *J Small Anim Pract* 1972; **13**: 425–437.

## 188–190: Questions

**188** What nerve and spinal cord segments are being tested? How do you interpret the results of this test?

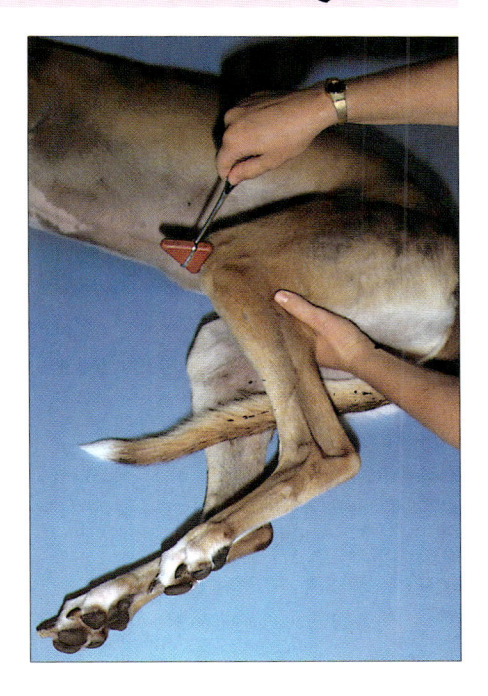

**189** Which of the following are recommended for maintenance therapy of epilepsy in cats? You may choose more than one answer.
a) Primidone.
b) Phenobarbitone.
c) Diazepam.
d) Phenytoin.

**190** A four-year-old German shepherd dog is being treated for idiopathic epilepsy. Therapy with phenobarbitone (3 mg/kg, twice daily) was started three months ago. The seizures are not controlled well, but the dog does not appear to be suffering any side-effects from the medication. Because of poor seizure control (several seizures per week), you decide to submit serum for determination of phenobarbitone concentration.
i. At what time of day should the sample be obtained?
ii. What is the target range?

## 188–190: Answers

**188** The patellar reflex is mediated through the femoral nerve and the L4–L6 spinal cord segments. A lesion located in this reflex arc will cause a decreased or absent patellar reflex, depending on the severity of the lesion. A lesion in the motor pathways cranial to the L4 spinal cord segment will result in a normal or exaggerated reflex. The patellar reflex is the most, and possibly only, reliable stretch reflex in veterinary medicine. However, there is some variability in this reflex among dogs and it depends on the animal's level of anxiety. The clinician should be hesitant to declare that there is a lesion cranial to L4 based on a mildly exaggerated patellar reflex in the absence of other signs of an upper motor neuron lesion, such as ataxia or paresis. The clinician should also realise that denervation of the flexor muscles of the stifle will cause an exaggerated patellar reflex. This most commonly occurs with a lesion of the sciatic nerve or L6–S2 spinal cord segments, which will cause a weak or absent flexor reflex.

**189** Phenobarbitone (b) and diazepam (c) are considered the drugs of first choice for maintenance anticonvulsant therapy in cats. Phenobarbitone is given initially at 1–2 mg/kg twice daily. With long-term therapy, the oral dose of phenobarbitone may need to be increased to maintain effective serum concentrations. The target range is 10–40 µg/ml. Diazepam, at 0.5–1 mg/kg divided into three doses per day, is also effective although it may be associated with liver disease in cats. The use of other anticonvulsant drugs in cats is hampered by limited clinical experience.

**Reference**
Schwartz-Porsche D, Kaiser E. Feline epilepsy. *Probl Vet Med* 1989; **1**: 628–649.

**190 i.** The trough serum concentration should be determined by collecting a serum sample immediately before the next scheduled dose. Serum concentrations should be measured when steady-state concentration has been reached – that is, when the amount of drug administered equals the amount of drug eliminated. For phenobarbitone, steady-state concentration is reached 10–14 days after starting therapy or changing the dose.
**ii.** The target range for phenobarbitone in dogs is approximately 20–40 µg/ml. Although the target range is a useful guide, it is a statistical value derived from population studies. The target range should not be rigidly adhered to without considering the individual patient's degree of seizure control and side-effects.

## 191–193: Questions

**191** Regarding the dog in **Q190**, the trough serum concentration of phenobarbitone is 14.6 µg/ml. What is your next step in the management of this dog?

**192** Regarding the dog in **Q190** and **Q191**, six months later, after increasing the phenobarbitone dose several times, the seizures are still poorly controlled (four seizures per week and several episodes of status epilepticus). The owner reports that the dog is persistently lethargic. A trough serum concentration of phenobarbitone is 47.4 µg/ml. Other than mild depression, no abnormalities are detected on physical and neurological examination. What is your next step?

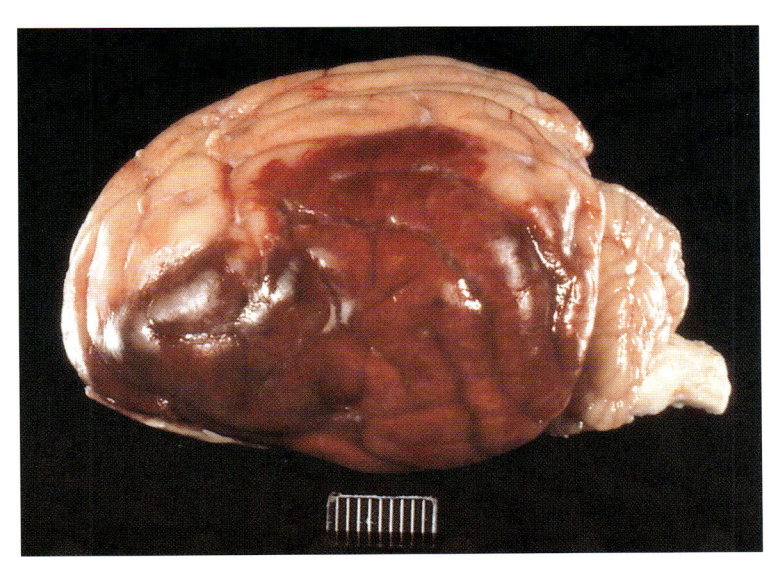

**193** This is a gross necropsy specimen (**above**) from a dog. What neurological deficits would be likely with this lesion?

# 191–193: Answers

**191** The serum concentration is below the target range and the seizures are not well controlled. The owner should be questioned to ensure the dog is actually receiving the prescribed dose of phenobarbitone. If compliance is good, the dose should be increased by 100%. This should achieve a serum concentration of approximately twice the current level. Two weeks after the change in dose, a trough serum concentration should be measured.

**Reference**
Forrester SD, Boothe DM, Troy GC. Current concepts in the management of canine epilepsy. *Compend Contin Educat Pract Vet* 1989; **11**: 811–820.

**192** The serum concentration exceeds the target range and the dog appears to be suffering from the side-effects (lethargy) of phenobarbitone therapy. If seizures are refractory to phenobarbitone therapy, the initial diagnosis should be re-evaluated. A physical and neurological examination should be performed. If any abnormalities are detected, further diagnostic evaluation is indicated, including CSF analysis and intracranial imaging. Also, the possibility of precipitating factors should be investigated. Drugs, such as phenothiazines, antihistamines, and some anthelmintics, may precipitate seizures in an epileptic dog. Concurrent diseases, emotional stress, and sleep deprivation may occasionally complicate management of epileptic animals.

If investigation does not detect an underlying disorder, combination therapy should be considered. The addition of potassium bromide (20–30 mg/kg, once daily) improves seizure control in many dogs with epilepsy refractory to phenobarbitone (Podell and Fenner, 1993). Because of its long elimination half-life, bromide does not reach steady-state concentration until 4–6 months. Side effects include polydipsia, sedation, and polyphagia. Serum bromide concentrations should be measured at one month and 4–6 months after initiating therapy. The target range is 1–2 mg/ml.

**Reference**
Podell M, Fenner WR. Bromide therapy in refractory canine idiopathic epilepsy. *J Vet Intern Med* 1993; **7**: 318–327.

**193** There is dark red discolouration of the lateral aspect of the left cerebral hemisphere. This is most likely due to haemorrhage. A lesion of the left cerebral hemisphere can cause decreased postural reactions on the right, blindness of the right visual field, decreased perception of cutaneous sensation on the right, and circling (usually to the left). Altered consciousness, abnormal behaviour, and seizures are also possible. Very large lesions, such as in this animal, may cause increased intracranial pressure. This may result in caudal tentorial herniation and signs of brainstem compression, including abnormal pupillary function, extensor rigidity, coma, abnormal respirations, and death.

**194–196: Questions**

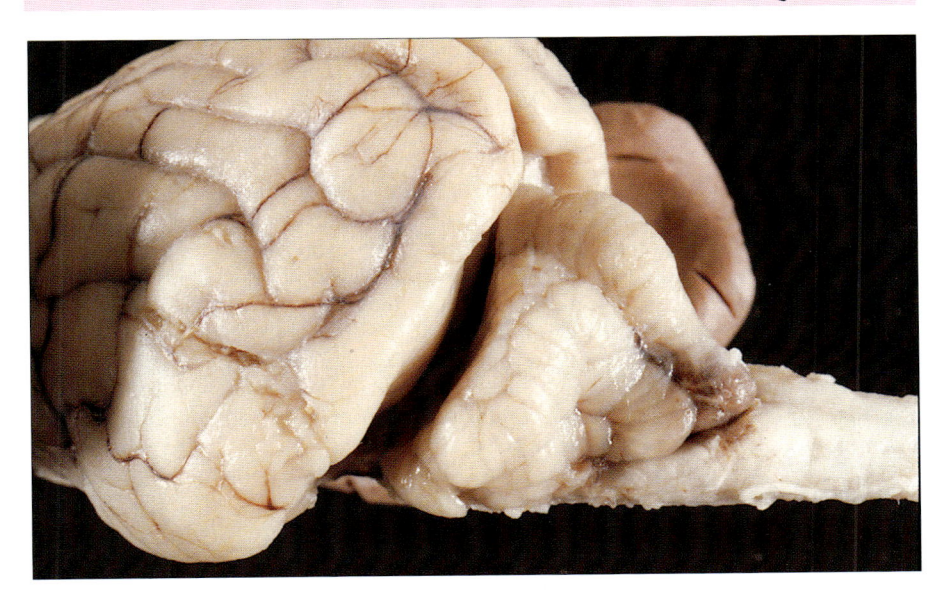

**194** What abnormality is evident in this illustration?

**195** What are the potential complications of myelography?

**196** Classify canine and feline spinal tumours, based on their location relative to the neural structures.

## 194–196: Answers

**194** Foramen magnum herniation – caudal displacement of the caudal cerebellar vermis through the foramen magnum. There is compression of the medulla oblongata and haemorrhage of the herniated portion of the cerebellum.

**195** Seizures occur infrequently following a myelogram. Neurological deterioration is rare following the procedure, but can occur. The incidence of complications with myelography is low when iohexol (Omnipaque®, Nycomed) is used.

Clearly, if the spinal puncture or injection technique is at fault, significant neurological damage may result. Injection of contrast into the central canal can occur in cisternal myelography; the effect on the patient varies, but is generally serious. Cardiovascular effects are usually seen and neurological deterioration is likely. Central canal injection in the lumbar spine is not usually associated with problems.

Lumbar myelography at sites cranial to L5/L6 may damage the lumbosacral intumescence and should not be performed.

It is not clear whether obtaining flexion, extension, or traction films during myelography can lead to neurological deterioration.

### Reference
Lewis DD, Hosgood G. Complications associated with the use of iohexol for myelography of the cervical vertebral column in dogs: 66 cases (1988–1990). *J Am Vet Med Assn* 1992; **200**: 1381–1384.
Wheeler SJ, Davies JV. Iohexol myelography in the dog and cat: a series of one hundred cases, and a comparison with metrizamide and iopamidol. *J Small Anim Pract* 1985; **26**: 247–256.

**196** See chart (**right**).

| Location | Type | Tumour |
|---|---|---|
| Extradural | Primary | Osteosarcoma |
|  |  | Fibrosarcoma |
|  |  | Chondrosarcoma |
|  |  | Lymphoma |
|  |  | Haemangiosarcoma |
|  |  | Myeloma |
|  | Secondary | Carcinoma |
|  |  | Sarcoma |
|  |  | Melanoma |
|  |  | Lymphoma |
| Intradural–Extramedullary | Primary | Meningioma |
|  |  | Nerve sheath tumours (schwannoma, neurofibroma, neurofibrosarcoma) |
|  |  | Neuroepithelioma |
|  |  | Sarcoma |
|  |  | Lymphoma |
|  | Secondary | Metastatic |
| Intramedullary | Primary | Glioma |
|  |  | Lymphoma |
|  |  | Haemangiosarcoma |
|  |  | Reticulosis |
|  | Secondary | Metastatic |

# 197–199: Questions

**197** What are these instruments (**right**) and what are they used for? Are there any limitations on their use in neurosurgery and, if so, why?

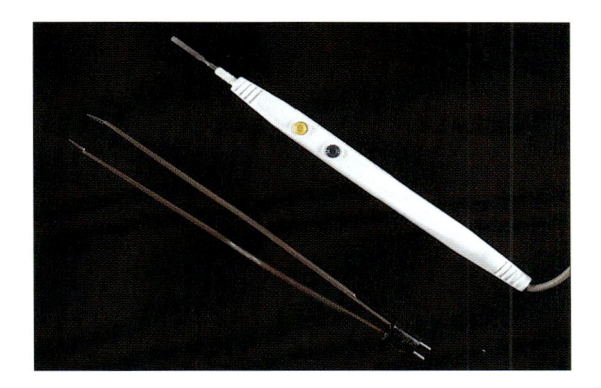

**198** This nine-year-old, mixed-breed dog is suffering from generalised weakness. The neurological examination reveals reduced CP (+1) in all limbs. The spinal reflexes are also depressed (+1). There is reduced muscle tone and mild muscle atrophy in the limbs. Sensation appears normal, as are all cranial nerve tests.
i. Localise the lesion.
ii. How would you investigate the patient further?

**199** This pigeon was presented because of a recent onset of neurological signs. The bird was disoriented and ataxic. There was paresis of the pelvic limbs and wings with increased muscle tone. The bird had intermittent opisthotonos. What is your primary diagnostic consideration?

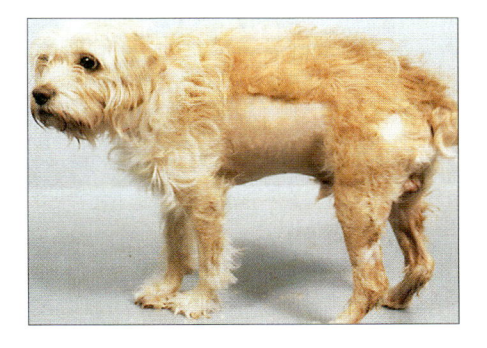

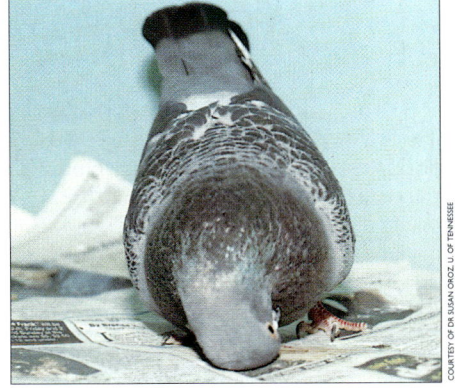

149

## 197–199: Answers

**197** These are electrosurgical instruments. The monopolar system (**above**) is used for coagulation and for incising tissues. Monopolar cautery must not be used in close proximity to nervous tissue, as the current travels through the patient and this can lead to tissue damage. Close to the nervous system, bipolar cautery (**below**) must be used, for example, in cauterising dural vessels.

**198 i.** The dog has generalised motor unit dysfunction, most likely a peripheral polyneuropathy.
**ii.** Haematology and biochemistry, including CK for evidence of muscle disease. (Pure muscle diseases do not typically result in CP deficits). Confirm the nature of the disorder with EMG and nerve conduction studies.

There are many causes of peripheral polyneuropathies. In a dog of this age, it is an acquired problem. Testing should include: • Serum biochemistry – some systemic diseases are associated with peripheral neuropathy, for example, hypoglycaemia. • Thyroid function – hypothyroidism may be related to peripheral neuropathy. • CSF collection and analysis – for evidence of nerve root disease. • *Toxoplasma* and *Neospora* titres. • Check for evidence of systemic cancer (peripheral neuropathy can be a paraneoplastic effect). • Immunological testing. • A thorough history to investigate exposure to toxins (lead, organophosphates).

Nerve biopsy should be considered, but only after an electrophysiological examination, and is probably best performed by a specialist. Despite extensive evaluations, many cases of peripheral neuropathy remain classified as 'idiopathic'.

### Reference
Duncan ID. Canine and feline peripheral polyneuropathies. In: Wheeler SJ (ed). *Manual of Small Animal Neurology*, 2nd edn. Cheltenham: BSAVA, 1995: 208–218.

**199** The neurological deficits are consistent with infection by paramyxovirus type-1. This virus is a neurotrophic, pigeon-adapted strain of Newcastle disease virus. Tonic paralysis of the wings, head tremor, and torticollis are common signs. A flaccid paralysis may also occur. The disease may be fatal or spontaneous recovery can occur. Diagnosis is by viral isolation. Other diagnostic considerations include nutritional deficiencies, toxins, and chlamydiosis.

### Reference
Bennett R.A. Neurology. In: Ritchie BW, Harrison GJ, Harrison LR (eds). *Avian Medicine: Principles and Application*. Lake Worth, USA: Wingers Publishing, 1994: 721–747.

# Index

All references are to question and answer numbers

Anaesthesia 48, 172
Analgesics 149, 150
Anisocoria 1
Antibiotics 27, 160, 183
Anticonvulsants 124, 157, 189
  complications 171
Aortic thromboembolism 141
Ataxia 118
Atlantoaxial subluxation 24, 25

Bladder function 82, 89, 92
Bone scintigraphy 131
Botulism 138, 161
Brachial plexus neoplasia 36, 102
Brachial plexus root avulsion 175
Brain, herniation 48, 87, 172, 194
  neoplasia 100, 120, 147
Brainstem auditory evoked potential 104
Bromide 157, 178
Brucellosis 58

Canine distemper encephalitis 83
Caudal cervical spondylomyelopathy 66, 167
Cerebellar, degeneration 9
  hypoplasia 93
Cerebrospinal fluid 19, 20, 29, 44, 125, 132, 162
Cervical disc disease 105
Computed tomography 4, 40, 48, 115, 151
Congenital disease 9
Coonhound paralysis 138
Corneal reflex 136
Corticosteroids 62, 148
Cranial nerve, V 43, 60, 95, 136
  VII 106, 163
  VIII 163
Crossed extensor reflex 158
Cryptococcus 153

Deafness 157
Decerebellate rigidity 184
Decubitus ulcer 73
Deep pain sensation 126
Degenerative myelopathy 91
Diabetic neuropathy 139
Disc degeneration 152
Discospondylitis 7, 8, 21, 26, 58, 131
Distal denervating disease 138

Electromyography 47
External ear canal 151

Facial nerve 106, 163, 186
Feline infectious peritonitis 185
Feline, leukaemia virus 98
  panleukopaenia virus 93
  spongiform encephalopathy 51, 52
Femoral nerve 188
Fibrocartilaginous embolisation 107, 134
Focal seizure 121
Foramen magnum herniation 194
Fucosidosis 9

Gastrointestinal ulceration 62
Generalised peripheral neuropathy 57
Giloma 115
Globoid cell leukodystrophy 176
Granulomatous meningoencephalomyelitis 18, 19, 132

Haemorrhage 193
Hepatic encephalopathy 78, 79, 80
Hepatoxicity 171
Hip dysplasia 90
Horner's syndrome 1, 45, 154, 163
Hydrocephalus 75, 140
Hypervitaminosis A 67
Hypoglycaemia 111
Hypokalemic polymyopathy 159
Hypomyelination 9, 181
Hypothyroidism 112

Iliac thrombosis 141
Incontinence 53, 82
Instrumentation 11, 49, 197
Insulinoma 111
Intervertebral disc disease 152
Ischaemic, encephalopathy 114
  myelopathy 107
  neuromyopathy 141
Ivermectin 127

Laryngeal paralysis 166
Localisation, brainstem 86
  cerebellum 93
  forebrain 39, 64, 113, 119
  lumbosacral intumescence 134
  multifocal 18, 33, 83
  peripheral neuropathy 138
  spinal 41, 81, 101, 107
  vestibular 83
Lower motor neuron 42
  diffuse 14
  disease 61
Lumbosacral disease 71, 130
Lymphoma 162
  spinal 98, 101

151

Magnetic resonance imaging 71, 147, 172
Mannitol 84
Masticatory muscle myositis 68
Megaesophagus 15
Menace response 10, 110
Meningioma 65, 142
Meningitis 26, 30, 133, 183
Methylprednisolone 81, 146
Metoclopramide 127
Metronidazole 127
Micturation 82, 89
Monoparesis, pelvic limb 94, 96
  thoracic limb 102, 175
Multiple cartilaginous exostoses 31
Muscular dystrophy 9, 182
Myasthenia gravis 15, 16, 169
Myelomalacia 63, 187
Mycoses, blastomycosis 28, 29
  cryptococcosis 153
Myelography 12, 44, 107, 174, 195
Myeloma 13

Narcolepsy 173
Nasopharyngeal polyp 6
Neoplasia 4, 12, 13, 26, 43, 65, 74, 100, 101, 102, 120, 123, 147, 177, 196
  chemotherapy 116
  nasal 120
Neosporosis 41
Nerve biopsy 57
Neuroepithelioma 74
Neurosurgery 160
Non-steroidal anti-inflammatory drugs 62

Optic neuritis 179, 180
Organophosphorous insecticides 127, 170
Ototoxicity 104

Patellar reflex 188
Pelvic fracture 23
Perineal reflex 161
Peripheral, nerve trauma 163
  neuropathy 47
Phenobarbitone 54, 85, 124, 190, 191
Pigeon, paramyxovirus 199
Pituitary adenoma 76, 77
Polyneuropathy 138, 139, 198
Portosystemic shunt 79, 80
Potassium bromide 157
Progressive, axonopathy 9
  myelomalacia 63, 187
Pug encephalitis 33, 34
Pupillary light reflex 35, 119, 155

Rabies 88
Radial nerve 55, 168
Radiation 37, 77, 100, 115
Radiology 22, 81
Rickettsial infection 129

Sacrocaudal trauma 92
Saphenous nerve 72
Schiff–Sherrington sign 56
Sciatic nerve 94, 96
Scotty cramp 99
Seizures 87, 85, 111, 124, 142, 157
  treatment 190, 191, 192
Spina bifida 17
Spinal cord trauma 146
Spinal disease, prognosis 126
Spinal needle 70
Spine neoplasia 4, 12, 13, 101, 196
Spondylosis 27, 137
Squamous cell carcinoma 151
Status epilepticus 38, 85, 144
Subdural haematoma 39, 40
Sudden acquired retinal degeneration 156
Surgery 11, 49, 160, 197
  cervical spine 143
  post-operative complications 73

Tetanus 103
Therapeutic drug monitoring 54
Thiamine deficiency 164
Thoracolumbar disc disease 2, 3, 22
  complications 62
Tibial nerve 165
Tick paralysis 14, 138
Toxicosis 127, 170
Transitional vertebrae 130
Trauma 23, 30, 56, 69, 81, 82, 86, 87, 146
Tremors 108, 109
Triceps reflex 168
Trigeminal, nerve 43, 95
  neuritis 95
Tumour 36, 37, 115
Tympanic bulla 5

Ultrasonography, brain 140
Upper motor neuron 42
Uretheral pressure profile 53

Vertebral, anomaly 32
  fracture 146
  osteomyelitis 26
  osteosarcoma 123
Vestibular syndrome 45, 46, 163, 177

Wobbler's syndrome 66, 167